THE GLUTEN-FREE COOKBOOK
FOR FAMILIES

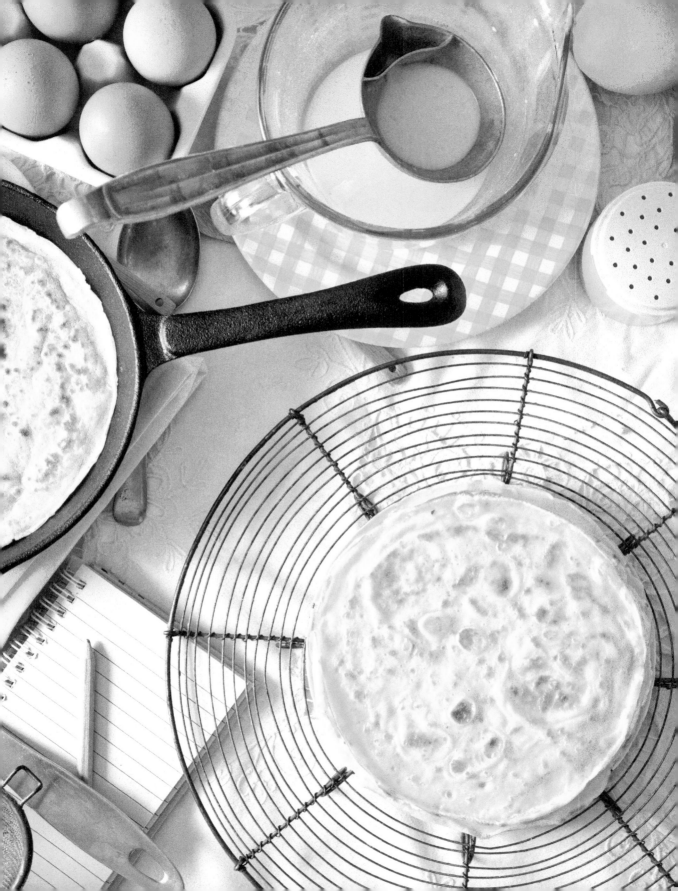

The GLUTEN-FREE COOKBOOK for Families

HEALTHY RECIPES IN 30 MINUTES OR LESS

PAMELA ELLGEN

ROCKRIDGE
PRESS

Photography © 2016 Offset/The Picture Pantry/Alanna Taylor-Tobin, cover (top right); Stocksy/Rachel Dewis, p.2; Stockfood/Gräfe & Unzer Verlag/Jörn Rynio, p.9; Ellie Baygulov/Stocksy, p.10; Shutterstock/Dani Vincek, p.15; Stockfood/Komar, cover (top left) and p.28; Stockfood/Louise Lister, p.54; Stockfood/Gräfe & Unzer Verlag/Wolfgang Schardt, p.78; Stockfood/George Seper, p.100; Stockfood/Geoff Fenney, cover (bottom right), spine and p.120; Stockfood/Andrew Young, p.154; Stocksy/Martí Sans, cover (bottom left) and p.184; Stockfood/Gareth Morgans, p.210; Stockfood/People Pictures, p.226.

ISBN: Print 978-1-62315-784-5 | eBook 978-1-62315-785-2

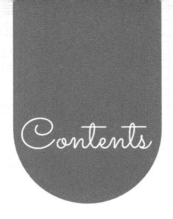

Contents

FOREWORD

Pamela Ellgen's *Gluten-Free Cookbook for Families* is just what the doctor ordered! When first diagnosed with celiac disease 23 years ago, I had never heard the phrase "gluten free," nor even known what gluten was. My doctor told me avoiding gluten completely—the only treatment for celiac disease—was going to be a challenge, but I was relieved to finally have an answer to years of unexplained symptoms. I soon learned, though, just how difficult the diet could be without proper nutritional guidance and a collection of tried-and-true recipes that were truly gluten free, tasty, and wholesome.

I started Beyond Celiac (formerly the National Foundation for Celiac Awareness), a nonprofit patient advocacy organization, in 2003 to increase the paltry 3 percent celiac disease diagnosis rate, to make gluten-free food safe and accessible to those who need it most, and to advance research. At the time there were no national organizations educating the public about the symptoms, the prevalence, and the genetic nature of celiac disease. I had suffered for years because my celiac disease went undetected by doctors, and I knew sharing this information would be essential to help more people like me get proper diagnosis and treatment.

Once diagnosed, navigating the gluten-free diet was tricky. There were few gluten-free products in grocery stores, and I rarely found individual ingredients, like gluten-free flours, to use in cooking. Having a cookbook packed with creative, appetizing recipes for every meal, such as those found in *The Gluten-Free Cookbook for Families*, would have made my transition to the gluten-free diet much easier.

Today options abound for gluten-free eating. Despite this, an air of mystery still surrounds the diet. Most of us did not eat this way growing up or learn to cook gluten-free meals, so many people aren't really sure where to begin.

Pamela's cookbook takes the mystery out of gluten-free cooking just as much as it infuses flavor into it. You'll find a variety of delicious recipes that appeal to all tastes and take less than 30 minutes to make. You'll also find a helpful guide to using different gluten-free flours, tips for eating in restaurants, and suggested menus for special occasions.

It takes a veteran of the gluten-free diet to include the diversity of tastes and ingredients found here. I was delightfully surprised to see recipes for sauces and marinades, knowing that purchased versions are frequent, hidden sources of gluten.

Having this comprehensive cookbook will prove a lifesaver whether you have a medical requirement to eat gluten free because of celiac disease, non-celiac gluten sensitivity, or a wheat allergy, or because you simply feel better eating this way due to other conditions. This cookbook contains recipes that take the guesswork out of cooking deliciously and filling your belly nutritiously.

Most of all, I was impressed by the thoughtful touches Pamela includes in the cookbook. She takes the time to define the different medical conditions that require a gluten-free diet, and she makes sure that her recipes accommodate other dietary needs that can to go along with a gluten-free diet. The recipes include substitution tips for the top eight food allergens (like dairy, tree nuts, and soy), and many recipes are appropriate for vegetarian and vegan diets.

Cooking and eating gluten-free food doesn't mean cooking and eating taste-free food. *The Gluten-Free Cookbook for Families* is proof of that.

—**ALICE BAST**

ABOUT THE FOREWORD CONTRIBUTOR

Alice Bast is the founder and CEO of Beyond Celiac, a national patient advocacy organization dedicated to serving people with celiac disease. Diagnosed after a decade-long search for answers to her life-interrupting symptoms, Bast founded Beyond Celiac in 2003, then known as the National Foundation for Celiac Awareness, to ensure that others do not suffer for years without answers the way she did. Today, Beyond Celiac serves over 2 million people through its robust social media presence and comprehensive website, www.BeyondCeliac.org.

INTRODUCTION

When I brought my second child, Cole, home from the hospital, life was pure bliss. He nursed contentedly. We enjoyed long naps while my husband stayed home from work to care for our older son, Brad. Our friends from church brought us endless meals. It was everything a new parent could hope for.

Well, it *was* everything we could hope for. At about six weeks old, Cole began to cry for hours at a time. No shushing or snuggling or bundling seemed to help. We took him on long drives throughout the city, hoping the car would lull him to sleep. We tried loud music, soft music, homeopathic drops for gas and upset stomach. Nothing seemed to work.

The doctor said my diet had nothing to do with his behavior. It was colic, it was natural, and it would eventually pass. I couldn't wait that long.

Finally, in tearful desperation, I called a family friend who is a lactation consultant. She encouraged me to eliminate wheat, dairy, and soy from my diet because the proteins in those foods could pass through my breast milk and possibly be the cause of Cole's distress. I gulped. No more triple-cream Brie cheese? No more crunchy French baguettes? I worried that I would miss out on some of my favorite foods. But, for the sanity of the whole family, it was worth a try.

Within a few days, we had a new baby. He was alert and relaxed during his waking times and slept peacefully during naps and at night. The change was undeniable, and we were beyond grateful.

However, now I had a new challenge on my hands. How could I cook meals that satisfied these new stringent dietary parameters without spending all day reading ingredient labels or cooking everything from scratch? To make matters more complicated, my husband, Rich, observed a mostly vegetarian diet, occasionally eating fish.

During that time, I tried nearly every gluten-free and dairy-free product on the market. Reading the nutrition labels was shocking—the first ingredient in most was sugar! How could that possibly be a healthy alternative? I also experimented with gluten-free baking but relied heavily on processed starches and gums. Eventually, working with foods that were naturally gluten-free proved to be the easiest, healthiest, and most sustainable option.

Throughout the process, I found that a gluten-free diet had a profound effect on my health. Food cravings disappeared, I easily lost the pregnancy weight, and I saw other long-term health concerns resolve naturally.

Fast-forward two years. During a parent–teacher conference with my older son's kindergarten teachers, they expressed concern at his inability to sit still or pay attention. They couldn't outright suggest a diagnosis or label, but the implications were clear to me. I decided to try dietary solutions before pursuing a medical diagnosis and medication. We put Brad on a gluten-free diet and within a week,

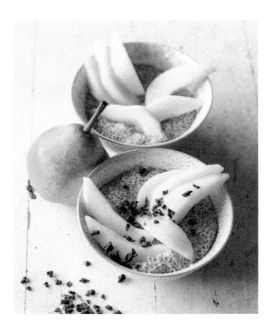

his teachers observed a change in him. He was calmer and more focused. Even more profound was that other seemingly unrelated health issues cleared up.

A gluten-free diet is now simply part of our family's daily life. Rich still eats wheat, but our home is stocked with naturally gluten-free foods and is free from the temptation of wheat-based snacks in the cupboard or the danger of the errant wheat crumbs in the toaster. Over the years, I've found simple, healthy, budget-friendly solutions to meet our dietary needs. Even better, we eat a wider variety of whole foods and enjoy plenty of decadent treats so the kids rarely feel deprived.

I hope that through this book, I can share everything I have learned from transitioning my family to a gluten-free diet. You can avoid the pitfalls I encountered and reap all the delicious rewards of a gluten-free diet, not only for you but for your entire family. The recipes in this book are quick and easy, include minimal sugar, and are naturally gluten-free or made with healthy substitutions for wheat products, such as whole-grain or nut-based flours. Because they have been helpful to us, I have also included recipes that are dairy-free, egg-free, vegetarian, and in line with other dietary preferences which may be helpful to you and your family.

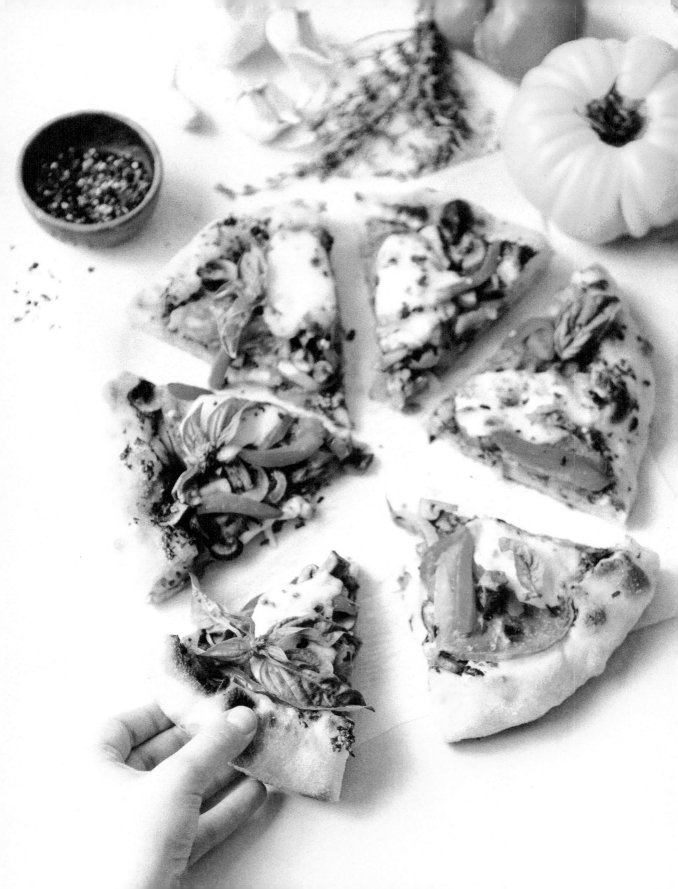

CHAPTER
One

HEALTHY GLUTEN-FREE LIVING
for Busy Families

Until recently, it seemed that only individuals with celiac disease or a rare handful of people in the natural health community went gluten-free. However, with books such as *Wheat Belly* and *Grain Brain* becoming bestsellers, and the rate of celiac diagnoses increasing, more and more people are turning to a gluten-free diet to address their health concerns. I am often surprised by the number of families I meet who follow a gluten-free diet. The need for a healthy approach to gluten-free cooking is more important than ever!

Is gluten-free synonymous with healthy? Not necessarily. Like any diet, there are healthy and not-so-healthy approaches. A gluten-free diet laden with processed foods, refined starches, and sugar—the foods that typically fill the gluten-free section of your supermarket—is not healthy or cheap.

A better approach is a diet that's *naturally* gluten-free. Ever seen gluten-free lettuce? How about gluten-free chicken? Of course you have. Foods that don't have a nutrition label typically don't have gluten in them, unless, of course, they're one of the four grains that contain the protein: wheat, barley, rye, and triticale. Shopping the perimeter of the grocery store generally keeps you in the naturally gluten-free section. These whole foods form the basis of the recipes in this book.

Initially, embarking on a gluten-free diet can be stressful and time consuming. After all, grain formed the basis of the USDA food pyramid for years, and wheat was, and still is, the most widely consumed grain in the United States. My hope is that this book will provide you with simple, easy, and quick recipes that satisfy both your dietary needs and your palate.

GLUTEN-RELATED DISORDERS

Gluten contains the proteins glutenin and gliadin. Gluten is found in several grains, including wheat, barley, rye, and triticale. Unless they're certified gluten-free, oats also contain gluten because they are processed on the same equipment as gluten-containing grains or grown near them.

There are three primary conditions associated with wheat and gluten:

1. CELIAC DISEASE

2. NONCELIAC GLUTEN SENSITIVITY

3. WHEAT ALLERGY

Celiac Disease

Celiac disease is a serious autoimmune disorder in which the immune system attacks the lining of the small intestine in response to gluten proteins. Any amount of gluten can trigger a reaction and subsequent damage. Therefore, a lifelong avoidance of gluten-containing foods is essential for people diagnosed with celiac disease.

The disease is underdiagnosed, meaning many people who have the disorder are not aware of it. It may or may not present outward symptoms, such as abdominal pain, joint pain, gastrointestinal problems, fatigue, malnutrition, weight loss, itching and rashes, and delayed growth. The disorder often runs in families, so if a parent, child, or sibling has celiac disease, it is worth seeing a doctor to evaluate your risk for the disease—especially if you have any of the symptoms listed previously. Long-term risks include the development of other autoimmune disorders, infertility and miscarriage, intestinal cancers, and neurological conditions.

Nonceliac Gluten Sensitivity

Nonceliac gluten sensitivity, sometimes referred to as NCGS, involves a reaction to gluten proteins without damage to the lining of the small intestine. It has been observed in clinical settings as early as 1980. However, NGCS has been slow to gain acceptance in the medical community as a legitimate condition because specific biomarkers are difficult to pinpoint and diagnostic criteria aren't agreed upon.

Symptoms of nonceliac gluten sensitivity include those present in celiac disease, such as abdominal pain, diarrhea, constipation, nausea, vomiting, muscle and joint pain, brain fog, migraines, numbness and tingling, rashes and itching, fatigue, and mental health conditions.

If you have symptoms of nonceliac gluten sensitivity and have ruled out celiac disease and a wheat allergy, you may opt to try a gluten-free diet for a period of time (usually two to four weeks) until symptoms subside, and then reintroduce gluten to establish whether your symptoms reemerge.

Wheat Allergy

A wheat allergy involves an allergic reaction to any one of the numerous proteins found in wheat. It is distinctly different from celiac disease, in which the reaction happens in the small intestine.

Symptoms of a wheat allergy include swelling, rashes and itching, hives, nasal congestion, headache, difficulty breathing, abdominal cramps, nausea, vomiting, diarrhea, and anaphylaxis. It is important to receive a proper medical diagnosis if you suspect a wheat allergy. Anaphylaxis is an acute, life-threatening condition that requires immediate medical attention.

A wheat allergy does not require abstinence from other gluten-containing grains, such as barley, rye, triticale, and oats, making it less restrictive than a completely gluten-free diet. Unlike celiac disease, a childhood wheat allergy may be outgrown by age three to five.

Other Common Food Sensitivities

Wheat is one of the top eight allergens, which include peanuts, tree nuts, fish, shellfish, eggs, milk, and soy. Allergies to these seven other allergens may accompany a wheat allergy. With this in mind, many recipes in this book are naturally allergen-free, or can be made so with a substitution or two, and are marked "Allergen-Free" where applicable.

Reactions to dairy are particularly common among people who have nonceliac gluten sensitivity. Because of this, most recipes in this book are free from dairy and are marked "Dairy-Free" where applicable.

Damage to the lining of the small intestine may also occur without celiac disease and result in what is indelicately referred to as "leaky gut syndrome." The condition causes the walls of the small intestine to allow food proteins to escape into the

The MICROBIOME and YOUR DIGESTIVE HEALTH

Your gut is home to trillions of bacteria, viruses, and fungal organisms—and that's a good thing! These organisms, collectively referred to as the microbiome, help you digest food, regulate metabolism, moderate your immune system, quell inflammation, remove toxins, and ensure efficient elimination. They also play a significant role in maintaining a healthy weight.

A proliferation of "bad" bacteria due to chronic stress, the overuse of antibiotics, or a diet full of refined carbohydrates will result in an imbalanced microbiome. So, too, will inadequate "good" bacteria due to eating a diet without much fiber or probiotics.

Restoring and fostering a healthy microbiome involves eating a diet with lots of fiber-rich produce, legumes, nuts, seeds, and whole grains, as well as prebiotic foods in the form of fermentable carbohydrates to feed the good bacteria, and probiotic-rich fermented foods to supplement the good bacteria. The good news is these foods are naturally gluten-free, and many are also vegan and free of the top eight allergens.

Unfortunately, many people with celiac disease continue to experience gastrointestinal symptoms due to an imbalanced gut microbiome even after they eliminate gluten. A study published in 2003 in the *American Journal of Gastroenterology* found that women with celiac disease experienced greater indigestion, constipation, and abdominal pain despite adherence to a gluten-free diet. Researchers noted this could be an effect of the gluten-free diet, which can be high in easily digestible starches.

Another study published in the same journal found a high prevalence of small intestine bacterial overgrowth (SIBO) in celiac patients who continued to experience gastrointestinal symptoms despite following a gluten-free diet. Treatment for SIBO involves the antibiotic rifaximin, which cleared up symptoms in all patients treated in the study. Drug-free

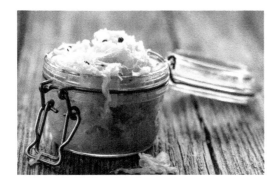

treatment options include the Specific Carbohydrate Diet, which excludes starches. It is similar to (but stricter than) the Paleo Diet. The low-FODMAP diet may also alleviate symptoms of a disrupted microbiome.

PREBIOTIC FOODS

Prebiotic foods contain fermentable fibers that pass through the digestive tract undigested and feed the healthy bacteria in the colon. Examples include almonds, asparagus, bananas, beans, beets, blueberries, bok choy, broccoli, cabbage, cashews, cauliflower, cherries, chickpeas, corn, fennel, garlic, leafy greens, lentils, mangos, nectarines, onions, peas, pistachios, plantains, polenta, pomegranate, and sweet potatoes.

PROBIOTIC FOODS

Probiotic foods contain live, active cultures that increase the population of healthy bacteria in the gastrointestinal tract. Examples include kefir, kimchee, kombucha, miso, raw honey, sauerkraut, gluten-free soy sauce, tempeh, and yogurt.

YOUR GUT HEALTH

I wrote a book devoted to recipes for gut health called *The Microbiome Cookbook*. The perspective I developed working on that book has contributed to the development of recipes for this book. Two additional cookbooks devoted to fermented foods include *Home Fermentation* and *DIY Fermentation* by Katherine Green.

blood stream, where they cause a wide array of symptoms, including those present in nonceliac gluten sensitivity. Leaky gut may also contribute to the development of food allergies.

FODMAP Sensitivity

FODMAP is an acronym that denotes fermentable carbohydrates, including wheat, some dairy products, many fruits, and a wide array of vegetables. It stands for fermentable oligosaccharides, disaccharides, monosaccharides, and polyols. People with gastrointestinal symptoms of nonceliac gluten sensitivity often find relief by following a low-FODMAP diet. In fact, the typical replacements for wheat flour found in many processed gluten-free products are high in these fermentable carbohydrates, resulting in even worse gastrointestinal symptoms. If you suspect sensitivity to FODMAP foods, definitely check out a cookbook devoted to low-FODMAP cooking. Just note that a low-FODMAP diet is a temporary solution and actually shouldn't be followed for a prolonged period.

INTEGRATING HEALTHY HABITS INTO BUSY LIVES

I know from personal experience how challenging it can be to cook healthy meals that satisfy the dietary preferences of the entire family while maintaining a reasonable food budget—it's a tall order. And, although I love spending time in the kitchen, I also love finding shortcuts to healthy meals so I can spend that extra time playing with my kids or simply enjoying the meal.

Here are ten tips that have worked for me and my family:

1. **Plan meals ahead of time.** I keep a list of my family's favorite meals and add to it when I find recipes we all enjoy. When it is time to plan each week's menu, I reach for that list first for most of the meal ideas, and then use cookbooks, magazines, or the farmers' market to inspire one or two new recipes each week. After that, I find I can do just one grocery shopping trip for the week and have healthy, fresh foods all week long. I also post the list of dinners on the refrigerator, and then we pick and choose based on the shelf life of produce or whatever we're feeling like that day.

2. **Keep it simple.** Pick recipes that involve five or fewer ingredients, or those that can be made in one pot. Also, look for recipes that don't require you to "transform" the ingredient. For example, peach chutney is delicious, but a simple uncooked peach salsa is even easier and saves you 30 minutes of cooking time.

3. **Build tradition into your weekly routine.** For a long time, we enjoyed family pizza night every Friday. When summer rolled around, it became family grill night. The more meals you can put on autopilot, the easier life will be. Other options include Tuesday taco night, meatless Mondays, and breakfast for dinner any night. Just pick the foods your family loves and set up a standing date every week.

4. **Get a jump-start on lunch prep.** I typically grocery shop on Fridays or early Saturday mornings. This gives me the entire weekend to leisurely prepare foods for the kids' lunches. I like to mix up a big batch of trail mix, clean and cut carrots and celery, and make a batch or two of gluten-free cookies. It makes the weekday morning rush much more manageable! I recently invested in lunch boxes with resealable individual compartments—no more wasted sandwich bags or leaking containers.

5. **Make the bulk bins your new best friend.** Chickpeas, lentils, 10-bean soup, and other bulk dried legumes make inexpensive, healthy, and filling meals. They do require a bit of forethought to presoak, but the cost is pennies on the dollar compared to canned beans.

6. **Keep healthy snacks on hand.** We have a large fruit bowl that is typically overflowing with bananas—my guys' go-to snack—and whatever else happens to be in season. Roasted nuts, blanched green beans, sliced carrots, and hard-boiled eggs are all great snack options.

7. **Keep a few processed snacks on hand.** While I love to cook whole-food ingredients from scratch, sometimes it's nice just to have a few relatively healthy gluten-free snacks I don't have to do anything to except open the bag. I choose those without added sugar and with as few ingredients as possible. Some of our family favorites include gluten-free pretzels, popcorn, Lärabars, dried fruit, and root vegetable chips.

8. **Make it once; eat it twice.** It takes much less effort to make one double batch of a recipe than to make it twice, especially with foods that require minimal preparation. For example, the Quinoa Fruit Salad recipe (page 32) can be prepared in fewer than five minutes if you cook a double batch of quinoa for dinner and use the leftovers to make the next day's breakfast. Enjoy the second batch as leftovers or freeze it and enjoy it the following week.

9. **Enlist your family's help.** When kids are very young, it's easier to do everything yourself, but once they're about five years old, they can contribute to meal preparation by setting the table and clearing plates. Slightly older kids can be trusted to clean lettuce, prepare salads, and cut vegetables.

10. **Stock prepared gluten-free dinner options.** It might seem counterintuitive for a cookbook to encourage you to purchase prepared gluten-free foods, but having a "just in case" meal on hand in the freezer or cupboard is a lifesaver. Some days it's 5 p.m. and the last thing I want to do is defrost a piece of fish or scrounge around the pantry to come up with a complete meal. Dinners out are expensive, and I get tired of checking and rechecking with restaurant servers about the possibility of gluten in my food. Trader Joe's sells some delicious gluten-free prepared meals. The vegetarian and/or healthy section of the frozen foods aisle at traditional grocery stores also offers some good gluten-free options, such as frozen veggie burritos and gluten-free pizza. Whole Foods is also an option; while it is expensive, it costs less than takeout or dining out.

When you're shopping for quick and easy gluten-free foods to prepare or to eat as snacks, you'll want to get comfortable remembering the following tips. With practice, running through these pointers as you browse the aisles will become second nature, and you'll be able to get through your grocery list faster.

Choose naturally gluten-free foods.

Many foods are naturally gluten free, so they may not feature a "gluten-free" label, but they're naturally free from the protein. Think carrots, white rice, salmon, or ground turkey.

Look for the allergen warning.

When products contain wheat or another top 8 allergen, labeling laws in the United States require it to be declared on the package. Although this can help you rule out the presence of wheat, the food may still contain gluten.

The FDA has standardized what "gluten-free" means on a food label, though it is not mandatory for companies to use. If a company does choose to label food as "gluten-free," "free of gluten," "no gluten," or "without gluten," then FDA regulations hold them accountable for ensuring that the food adheres to a gluten limit of less than 20 parts per million (ppm) for that food.

Know the code.

Gluten is rarely listed as an ingredient. Instead, look for words that indicate the presence of gluten-containing grains: semolina, spelt, durum, barley, malt, rye, and gram.

Enlist the help of an app.

Smartphone or tablet apps such as ipiit The Food Ambassador and Fooducate Allergy & Gluten Free Diet Tracker allow you to scan the bar code on popular foods to screen for the presence of gluten and other common allergens.

THE JOY OF GLUTEN-FREE COOKING

One of the greatest joys for me in gluten-free cooking is knowing all the ingredients going into my kids' meals are healthy and, without a doubt, free from gluten. I feel a sense of empowerment and l relish those moments when my kids say, "Yes!" when they see their favorite gluten-free meal on their plate.

What Not to Eat (and Why)

The obvious sources of gluten are foods that contain wheat, barley, rye, and triticale. Different kinds of wheat are known by alternative names, including durum, emmer, semolina, spelt, farina, farro, graham, kamut, and einkorn. By law, any product that

NOT ALL *Substitutions* ARE CREATED *Equal*

There are myriad gluten-free options for replacing wheat flour in cooking. Some are better suited to specific tasks than others. Basically all must be combined with one or more gluten-free flours to yield desirable taste and texture in baking. Here are the pros and cons of some of the most widely used gluten-free flours.

INGREDIENT	DESCRIPTION	PROS	CONS
ALMOND FLOUR	Made from finely ground blanched almonds; grain-free	High protein, moderate fiber, low glycemic index	Dense, expensive
AMARANTH FLOUR	Made from ground amaranth grain	Whole grain, moderate fiber, moderate protein	Distinct nutty, malt flavor (may be a positive trait in some recipes)
ARROWROOT	Made from the starchy rhizome arrowroot; grain-free	Good texture in baked goods; thickening properties similar to cornstarch	Cannot be reheated for thickening sauces; high glycemic index, no fiber
BROWN RICE FLOUR	Made from stone-ground brown rice	Whole grain, moderate protein, moderate fiber; yields volume in baked goods	Grainy texture
COCONUT FLOUR	Made from defatted dried coconut; grain-free	High fiber, low carbohydrate; absorbs a large volume of liquid	Easy to overuse and yield dryness in baked goods

INGREDIENT	DESCRIPTION	PROS	CONS
GARBANZO BEAN/ FAVA BEAN FLOUR	Made from garbanzo beans and fava beans; grain-free	High fiber, high protein	Subtle, but distinct, flavor
GUAR GUM	Derived from ground guar beans	Used in very small quantities to mimic the elastic qualities of gluten and allow foods to rise properly	Easy to overuse, produces a gummy texture
MILLET FLOUR	Made from ground millet	Whole grain, moderate fiber, moderate protein; produces a fine crumb in baking	None
POTATO STARCH, NOT POTATO FLOUR	Made from high-starch potatoes; grain-free	Produces a tender, fine crumb in baking	High glycemic index, low nutritional value
SORGHUM FLOUR	Made from ground sorghum grain	Whole grain, moderate fiber, moderate protein	None
TAPIOCA FLOUR (STARCH)	Made from cassava root; grain-free	Thickening and gelling properties	High glycemic index, low nutritional value
XANTHAN GUM	A fine polysac-charide powder derived from fermentation	Used in very small quantities to mimic the elastic qualities of gluten and allow foods to rise properly	Easy to overuse, produces a gummy texture

contains wheat must list it clearly in the ingredients and/or specify it on the packaging. However, the other gluten-containing grains are not subject to the same regulations.

Foods that *typically include* these grains include, but are not limited, to:

- Baked goods
- Breads and pastries
- Brewer's yeast and malt
- Cereal and granola
- Crackers and cookies
- Croutons and bread crumbs
- Flour tortillas
- Pancakes and waffles
- Pasta and noodles
- Sauces and gravies
- Seitan

Foods that *sometimes* contain gluten include, but are not limited, to:

- Candy, which often contains wheat as a thickener or in the form of crisp pieces
- Cheesecake filling, sometimes thickened with wheat flour
- Cheese shreds, sometimes coated with wheat starch, must be labeled as "containing wheat" if so; read nutrition labels to verify
- Communion wafers, which are sometimes made with wheat flour
- French fries and hash browns are sometimes coated with wheat flour or fried in a deep fryer that has cooked other foods containing wheat
- Multigrain products, such as tortilla chips and cereals, which often contain wheat
- Packaged foods often contain wheat; read labels and consult manufacturers to verify
- Processed meats and meat substitutes, which sometimes contain gluten, especially vegetarian burgers
- Risotto, sometimes thickened with wheat flour
- Soup, often thickened with wheat flour
- Soy sauce, unless labeled "gluten-free," is made with wheat flour

Finding replacements for these foods has never been easier, but that doesn't mean all gluten-free alternatives are good for your health. Most gluten-free baked goods and snacks are filled with processed flours, such as white rice flour, tapioca flour (starch), arrowroot, and potato starch, which all have a higher glycemic index (greater impact on your blood sugar) than all-purpose white flour. Worse yet, many gluten-free cereals and baking mixes list sugar as the first ingredient, meaning it's the most prevalent.

Because rice is a common replacement for wheat in a gluten-free diet, overexposure to arsenic is a concern. A 2012 investigation conducted by *Consumer Reports* found high levels of arsenic in rice, especially brown rice, compared to other grains. While no safe level has been established for arsenic exposure, there is no federal limit on arsenic in foods. In this book, I use a whole-grain blend that includes some brown rice flour, but you can also use a completely grain-free flour blend using finely ground blanched almond flour.

Kitchen Equipment and Pantry Lists

An arsenal of basic kitchen tools makes cooking and baking easy and is helpful in your kitchen. You probably have most of these items already:

- Blender, high-speed
- Blender, immersion
- Candy thermometer
- Cast-iron skillet
- Coffee grinder for nuts
- Food processor with grater attachment
- Glass jars (various sizes) with lids
- Good-quality 14-inch skillet and 8-inch skillet with lids
- Good-quality chef's knife
- Hand mixer
- Measuring cups, liquid and dry
- Measuring spoons
- Meat thermometer
- Metal strainer
- Microplane grater
- Muffin tin (standard 12-cup)
- Parchment paper
- Pastry brush
- Pots with lids
- Rolling pin
- Rubber and metal spatulas
- Vegetable peeler
- Wire whisk
- Wooden spoon
- Zester

A few essential pantry items will also be helpful in preparing the recipes in this book:

Baking powder Buy aluminum-free, double-acting baking powder for best results. Most baking powder sold in the United States is already gluten-free because the active ingredients are suspended in cornstarch.

Baking soda You'll use this in some recipes that contain an acid for the soda to react with and create a rise in the food.

Gluten-Free FLOUR MIXES

Numerous flour companies offer gluten-free flour blends, some of which include gums to replicate the effects of gluten. With the exception of Bob's Red Mill, most flour blends that seek to replicate all-purpose wheat flour have a similarly poor nutritional profile. Here are some of the more popular brands of all-purpose flours and their ingredients.

Nutrition information reflects a ¼-cup serving.

Arrowhead Mills Organic Gluten-Free Heritage Blend All-Purpose Flour: organic sorghum flour, organic rice flour, organic tapioca flour, organic millet flour, organic buckwheat flour, organic inulin, xanthan gum; 130 calories, 3g protein, 3g fiber

Betty Crocker Gluten-Free Rice Flour Blend: rice flour, potato starch, tapioca flour (starch), guar gum, salt; 110 calories, 1g protein, 1g fiber

Bob's Red Mill All-Purpose Baking Flour: garbanzo bean flour, potato starch, tapioca flour (starch), whole-grain sweet white sorghum flour, fava bean flour; 100 calories, 3g protein, 3g fiber

Cup4Cup Original Multipurpose Flour: cornstarch, white rice flour, brown rice flour, milk powder, tapioca flour (starch), potato starch, xanthan gum; 100 calories, 2g protein, 0g fiber

King Arthur Gluten-Free Whole-Grain Flour Blend: sorghum, brown rice (rice flour, rice bran) amaranth, quinoa, millet, teff, tapioca flour; 110 calories, 2g protein, 0g fiber

Pamela's Products Flour Blend: brown rice flour, tapioca flour (starch), white rice flour, potato starch, sorghum flour, arrowroot starch, guar gum, sweet rice flour, rice bran; 110 calories, 1g protein, 1.5g fiber

You can also make your own gluten-free flour blend with a mixture of about 70 percent whole-grain flours and 30 percent starches. I use guar gum, but you can use xanthan gum if you prefer it.

Whole-Grain Gluten-Free Flour Blend

1 cup millet flour

1 cup sorghum flour

¾ cup brown rice flour

¾ cup potato starch

½ cup tapioca flour (starch)

1 tablespoon guar gum

Per Serving (1 cup): Calories 477; Total
Carbohydrates 103g; Sugar 1g; Total
Fat 4g; Saturated Fat 1g; Sodium 8mg;
Protein 10g; Fiber: 7g

If you prefer to purchase a premixed whole-grain flour blend, use the Arrowhead Mills Organic Gluten-Free Heritage Blend All-Purpose Flour or King Arthur Gluten-Free Whole-Grain Flour Blend. These commercial blends absorb more liquid than my gluten-free flour blend recipe, and you may need to add more liquid or slightly reduce the amount of flour called for in the recipes.

Measuring Flour

To get accurate amounts when measuring flour for a recipe, follow these steps:

1. Fluff the flour with a spoon.
2. Scoop the flour from its container into a dry measuring cup. Do not pack it or tap it to settle.
3. Scrape away the excess with the blunt side of a knife swept across the top of the measuring cup.

Butter Used in some recipes and should be unsalted.

Coconut oil This oil is useful for high-heat cooking because it has a high smoke point.

Extra-virgin olive oil This ingredient is used in all salad dressings in this book and, occasionally, for cooking.

Gluten-free flours and flour blends Essential for gluten-free baking and for making sauces and breading. If you are new to gluten-free cooking, buying several flours may induce some sticker shock. But, once you have them, you'll only need to replenish one or two at a time. I suggest you start with brown rice flour, millet flour, potato starch, sorghum flour, and tapioca flour (starch).

Gluten-free pasta This shelf-stable ingredient makes dinner easy to pull together at a moment's notice. I also enjoy purchasing fresh gluten-free pasta from specialty markets. It rivals the fresh wheat-flour pastas I used to make at home.

Gluten-free soy sauce, or tamari Useful in Asian cooking.

Quinoa Packed with protein and fiber, this is an excellent option for vegetarian dinners.

Red wine vinegar The ingredient I reach for most when making salad dressings and to add acidity to sauces. You can also use white wine vinegar or apple cider vinegar. Balsamic vinegar has a delicious, complex flavor, but should not be used as a substitute for red wine vinegar.

Rice, white and brown Both are useful for risotto and also make an easy gluten-free side dish.

Sea salt I use this in all recipes in this book. Kosher salt is an acceptable substitute. If you use regular table salt, reduce the amount of salt called for in each recipe by half, and then adjust to taste.

Shortening This ingredient is sometimes called for as a dairy-free and vegan alternative to butter. Choose a nonhydrogenated shortening. I prefer Spectrum Organic All-Vegetable Shortening.

Recipe Labels

Recipes include the following labels, where applicable, to help you navigate additional dietary restrictions and choose convenient options for your family's needs:

Allergen-Free contains none of the top eight allergens, which are wheat, dairy, egg, soy, peanuts, tree nuts, fish, or shellfish, or can easily be modified to exclude them.

Dairy-Free contains no cow's milk products.

Egg-Free contains no eggs.

Nut-Free contains no tree nuts or peanuts.

One Pot can be made in one dish, pot, pan, or container.

Slow Cooker Option can be made in a slow cooker.

Splurge-Worthy ingredients are more expensive than usual, but worth it for special occasions.

Vegan contains no meat, fish, dairy, eggs, or honey. These recipes are dairy-free and egg-free.

Vegetarian contains no meat or fish.

For each recipe, nutritional information is calculated by taking the total nutrition of a recipe and dividing it by the number of servings. When a recipe suggests a range of servings, the larger serving size was used to calculate the nutritional information. For example, if a recipe serves 4 to 6 people, the nutritional information was calculated based on 4 servings.

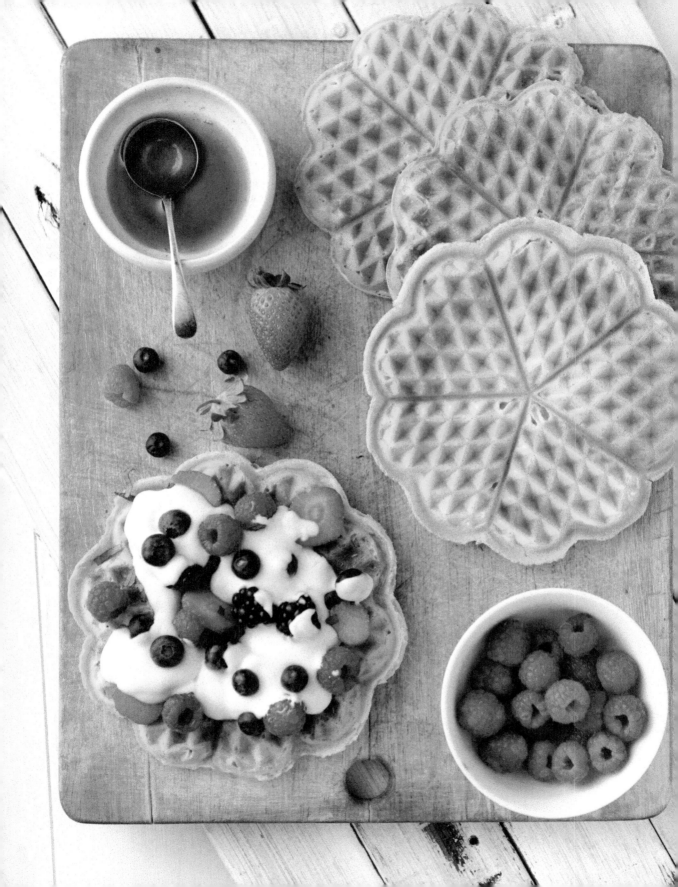

CHAPTER
Two

BREAKFAST

ALMOND BUTTER
Smoothie

SERVES 4 ° PREP TIME: 5 MINUTES

ONE POT
VEGAN

4 ripe bananas
2 cups unsweetened
  almond milk
½ cup roasted salted
  almond butter
Pinch sea salt
1 to 2 cups crushed ice

This is a breakfast recipe I could enjoy every day and be perfectly content. If you want extra protein, add a scoop of vanilla or chocolate protein powder. For a really chocolaty version, add 1 tablespoon of unsweetened cocoa powder.

1. In a blender, combine the bananas, almond milk, almond butter, and salt. Blend until smooth.

2. Add the ice based on desired thickness and blend until all the ice chunks are integrated and the smoothie is cold and thick.

INGREDIENT TIP For an extra-creamy and cool smoothie, use frozen bananas and omit the ice from the recipe. To freeze the bananas, peel them, cut them in slices, spread them out on a baking sheet, and place in the freezer until solid. Transfer to a covered container and store in the freezer.

PER SERVING Calories 318; Total Carbohydrates 34g; Sugar 14g; Total Fat 19g; Saturated Fat 2g; Sodium 140mg; Protein 9g; Fiber 5g

BASIC GREEN
Smoothie

SERVES 2 ° PREP TIME: 10 MINUTES

4 cups chopped fresh
  kale, tough ribs removed
1 cup roughly chopped
  fresh cilantro
½ cup roughly chopped
  fresh parsley
2 limes, peeled
1 orange, peeled
1 to 2 cups water
2 cups frozen pineapple

This smoothie has the perfect balance of sweet, tart, and herbaceous notes. Even my kids love it, which is a blessing because they're much less interested in kale salads. Use spinach in place of kale if that is what you have on hand.

1. In a blender, combine the kale, cilantro, parsley, limes, and orange. Add just enough water as needed to get the mixture moving. Blend until mostly smooth.

2. Add the frozen pineapple and blend until smooth.

INGREDIENT TIP To peel citrus quickly, cut off both ends of the fruit and stand it on one end. Use a sharp paring knife to cut away the peel and pith (the white underlayer). Swap the limes for lemons, if you prefer, but be sure to remove the seeds—unless you have a powerful high-speed blender.

PER SERVING Calories 219; Total Carbohydrates 55g; Sugar 26g; Total Fat 1g; Saturated Fat 0g; Sodium 73g; Protein 7g; Fiber 9g

QUINOA FRUIT SALAD

SERVES 4 ° PREP TIME: 1O MINUTES ° COOK TIME: 2O MINUTES
CHILL TIME: 2O MINUTES

ALLERGEN-FREE
NUT-FREE
ONE POT
VEGAN

1 cup quinoa, rinsed
  and drained
2 cups water
Pinch sea salt
Zest of 1 lime
Juice of 1 lime
2 cups green
  grapes, halved
1 cup fresh strawberries
1 cup fresh blueberries
4 fresh mint leaves,
  thinly sliced

While growing up, I remember my mom preparing many alternative grains for breakfast. Whenever she made millet, we would jokingly call it birdseed. Whatever you call it, eating whole grains for breakfast is healthy, because they are loaded with protein and complex carbohydrates. They also make a satisfying lunch.

1. In a medium pot over medium heat, combine the quinoa, water, and salt. Bring to a simmer and then reduce the heat to low. Cover and cook for about 20 minutes, until the quinoa is cooked through. Remove from the heat and fluff with a fork.

2. Stir in the lime zest and juice, grapes, strawberries, and blueberries. Chill for 20 minutes or until ready to serve.

3. Just before serving, stir in the mint leaves.

SERVING TIP You can prepare this dish the night before so it's ready to enjoy in the morning. Even better, if you're preparing quinoa for dinner, double the recipe and use the leftovers in this recipe for breakfast.

PER SERVING Calories 225; Total Carbohydrates 45g; Sugar 13g; Total Fat 3g; Saturated Fat 0g; Sodium 63g; Protein 7g; Fiber 6g

CHIA PUDDING

SERVES 4 ∘ PREP TIME: 5 MINUTES ∘ CHILL TIME: 25 MINUTES

ONE POT
VEGAN
MAKE ALLERGEN-FREE

2 cups unsweetened
  almond milk
⅔ cup chia seeds
2 tablespoons maple syrup
1 teaspoon vanilla extract
Sliced fresh pears,
  for serving
Cacao nibs, for
  garnish (optional)

When my husband and I discovered that professional surfer Kelly Slater enjoys chia pudding for breakfast, we were sold! Turns out chia seeds are a favorite of athletes and have been for millennia. The ancient Aztecs even called them "the running seed." They're packed with protein, fiber, and healthy omega-3 fats.

1. In a medium bowl, whisk the almond milk, chia seeds, maple syrup, and vanilla until thoroughly mixed. Cover and refrigerate for 25 minutes, or overnight.

2. Serve with sliced pears and garnish with cacao nibs (if using).

COOKING TIP Prepare this pudding the night before to save precious time during the morning rush.

SUBSTITUTION TIP Use rice milk to make this allergen-free.

PER SERVING Calories 228; Total Carbohydrates 35g; Sugar 16g; Total Fat 9g; Saturated Fat 1g; Sodium 7mg; Protein 5g; Fiber 13g

BANOFFEE PIE
Pudding Cups

SERVES 4 ∘ PREP TIME: 5 MINUTES

ONE POT
VEGAN

1 cup raw cashews
2 ripe bananas
½ cup brewed coffee
¼ cup coconut oil, melted
1 teaspoon vanilla extract
Pinch sea salt

Want dessert for breakfast? I sure do! These delicious little puddings are inspired by raw, vegan "cheese-cake" recipes and the British dessert banoffee pie. Because this version contains no refined sweetener, I feel completely comfortable serving it for breakfast. The amount of caffeine per serving is minimal but, if you're concerned about it, use decaf coffee.

1. In a blender, combine all the ingredients and purée until very smooth.

2. Evenly divide the mixture among 4 ramekins or small glass jars. Enjoy immediately or cover and refrigerate overnight for a firm texture.

INGREDIENT TIP Soaking the cashews ahead of time will improve their digestibility and make them easier to blend. Cover the raw cashews with several cups of fresh water and let sit at room temperature for 4 hours, or up to 24 hours in the refrigerator. Rinse thoroughly and drain. The water contains enzyme inhibitors and should be discarded.

PER SERVING Calories 370; Total Carbohydrates 25g; Sugar 9g; Total Fat 30g; Saturated Fat 15g; Sodium 65g; Protein 6g; Fiber 3g

CINNAMON RAISIN
Granola

MAKES 8 CUPS ∘ PREP TIME: 5 MINUTES ∘ COOK TIME: 25 MINUTES

VEGAN
MAKE ALLERGEN-FREE
MAKE NUT-FREE

6 cups gluten-free oats
1 cup sliced toasted
  almonds (optional)
¼ cup canola oil
¼ cup maple syrup
1 teaspoon vanilla extract
2 teaspoons ground
  cinnamon
⅛ teaspoon sea salt
1 cup raisins

I grew up enjoying this granola and now I make it for my kids. It is so much healthier than most breakfast cereals—even the gluten-free ones, which are still little more than refined grains coated in sugar and artificial colors.

1. Preheat the oven to 325°F.

2. In a large bowl, stir together the oats and almonds (if using).

3. In a large measuring cup, whisk the canola oil, maple syrup, vanilla, cinnamon, and salt. The ingredients will not emulsify, but do your best to combine them. Pour the liquid mixture over the oats and stir to coat them thoroughly.

4. Spread the oats over a baking sheet. Bake for 15 minutes. Use a spatula to stir the granola, so the mixture at the edges moves toward the center, and what was on the bottom is now on the top. Bake for 5 minutes more. Stir again. Bake for another 5 minutes, or until the mixture is golden brown.

5. Cool the mixture completely before stirring in the raisins. Store in a covered container in the pantry for up to 2 weeks.

SUBSTITUTION TIP To make this allergen-free and nut-free, omit the almonds. I prefer to bake with coconut oil because it has healthy fats that are easily used for energy. Use it in place of canola oil in this recipe, if you wish. Melted butter or ghee are delicious substitutions, if a vegan version is not needed.

PER SERVING Calories 188; Total Carbohydrates 32g; Sugar 9g; Total Fat 6g; Saturated Fat 1g; Sodium 19mg; Protein 4g; Fiber 4g

GRAIN-FREE
Granola

MAKES 5 CUPS ° PREP TIME: 5 MINUTES ° COOK TIME: 25 MINUTES

VEGAN

½ cup pitted
  Medjool dates
⅓ cup very hot water
¼ cup coconut oil, melted
2 teaspoons vanilla extract
⅛ teaspoon sea salt
1 cup walnuts
1 cup almonds
1 cup cashews
1 cup shredded
  unsweetened coconut
1 cup raisins

I have spent the past few years exploring Paleo cooking, including grain-free baking. This recipe is completely grain-free and has a similar texture to artisan granola. It is very filling, so a half-cup serving will easily keep me satisfied until lunch.

1. Preheat the oven to 350°F.

2. In a medium bowl, cover the dates with the hot water and soak for 5 minutes.

3. Add the coconut oil, vanilla, and salt. Transfer the date mixture to a blender, or use an immersion blender, and purée until mostly smooth.

4. In a food processor, combine the walnuts, almonds, and cashews. Pulse until coarsely chopped.

5. Add the coconut and pulse once or twice, just to integrate.

6. Pour in the date purée and pulse one or two more times, or stir by hand with a spatula.

7. Spread the mixture on a baking sheet and bake for 10 minutes.

8. Use a spatula to flip the nut mixture, trying to keep pieces intact as if they were cookies or bars, and then bake for 10 minutes more. Stir the mixture one more time and return it to the oven for 5 minutes. Remove the pan from the oven and stir in the raisins.

9. Cool completely before storing in a covered container in the refrigerator for up to 1 week.

SUBSTITUTION TIP This granola is naturally sweetened by the date purée. However, if dates are not easily available, use ½ cup of maple syrup instead.

PER SERVING Calories 357; Total Carbohydrates 27g; Sugar 16g; Total Fat 27g; Saturated Fat 9g; Sodium 29mg; Protein 8g; Fiber 16g

PANCAKES

SERVES 4 ° PREP TIME: 5 MINUTES ° COOK TIME: 1O MINUTES

NUT-FREE
VEGETARIAN
MAKE DAIRY-FREE

1 ½ cups Whole-Grain
   Gluten-Free Flour
   Blend (page 25)
1 tablespoon sugar
2 teaspoons aluminum-
   free, double-acting
   baking powder
¼ teaspoon sea salt
2 eggs
1 to 1 ½ cups milk
3 tablespoons canola oil
1 teaspoon vanilla extract

My kids love it when I make gluten-free pancakes. So, when I began testing recipes for this book, they were in heaven. I wanted to create a recipe that resembled traditional pancakes but without relying heavily on refined gluten-free flours and starches. My Whole-Grain Gluten-Free Flour Blend (page 25) is built on a combination of whole-grain sorghum, whole-grain millet, and whole-grain brown rice flours, with a small amount of potato and tapioca starches for improved texture and browning. I'm so glad to share this recipe with you!

1. In a large bowl, combine the flour blend, sugar, baking powder, and salt.

2. In a medium bowl, whisk the eggs, milk, canola oil, and vanilla. Pour the milk mixture into the flour mixture and whisk to break up any lumps. Add more milk, if needed, to get a thick but pourable batter.

3. Heat a large nonstick griddle or skillet over medium heat.

4. With a ¼-cup measuring cup, ladle the batter onto the hot griddle. Cook for 1 to 2 minutes until the edges are set and bubbles rise in the center of the pancakes. Flip and cook for another 1 to 2 minutes on the other side. Repeat with the remaining batter.

COOKING TIP Save time by preparing the dry ingredients ahead of time. Store in a covered container so you're ready to whip up a batch of pancakes any time.

SUBSTITUTION TIP To make this dairy-free, use nondairy milk.

PER SERVING Calories 357; Total Carbohydrates 45g; Sugar 8g; Total Fat 15g; Saturated Fat 3g; Sodium 194mg; Protein 11g; Fiber 1g

WAFFLES

SERVES 4 ° PREP TIME: 5 MINUTES ° COOK TIME: 20 MINUTES

NUT-FREE
VEGETARIAN
MAKE DAIRY-FREE

2 cups Whole-Grain
  Gluten-Free Flour
  Blend (Page 25)
1 tablespoon sugar
1 tablespoon aluminum-
  free, double-acting
  baking powder
¼ teaspoon sea salt
3 eggs
½ cup milk
½ cup (1 stick)
  butter, melted
1 teaspoon vanilla extract

I'm a little late to the waffle craze—but better late than never! These waffles make a delicious breakfast or can be served with Panfried Crispy Chicken (page 132) for a soul-food supper. The butter (or oil, if choosing the dairy-free option) in the batter produces a delicious, crispy waffle, but you can reduce it to ¼ cup if you prefer a lower fat version. Enjoy topped with mixed fresh berries, some crème fraîche (if dairy is not a concern), and a drizzle of maple syrup.

1. In a large bowl, combine the flour blend, sugar, baking powder, and salt.

2. In a medium bowl, whisk the eggs, milk, butter, and vanilla. Pour the milk mixture into the flour mixture, and whisk to break up any lumps. Add more milk, if needed, to get a thick but pourable batter.

3. Heat a waffle iron according the manufacturer's directions.

4. With a ¼-cup measuring cup, ladle the batter onto the hot waffle iron. Cook according to the waffle iron manufacturer's instructions.

5. Transfer to a heatproof plate in a warm oven until ready to serve. Repeat with the remaining batter.

COOKING TIP Save time by preparing the dry ingredients ahead of time. Store in a covered container so you're ready to whip up a batch of waffles any time.

SUBSTITUTION TIP To make this dairy-free, use nondairy milk.

PER SERVING Calories 511; Total Carbohydrates 54g; Sugar 5g; Total Fat 28g; Saturated Fat 16g; Sodium 348mg; Protein 12g; Fiber 2g

SUN-DRIED TOMATO AND EGG
Muffin Cups

SERVES 6 ∘ PREP TIME: 5 MINUTES ∘ COOK TIME: 15 MINUTES

NUT-FREE
VEGETARIAN
MAKE DAIRY-FREE

12 eggs
½ teaspoon sea salt
1 ½ cups shredded
  fresh spinach
½ cup minced oil-packed
  sun-dried tomatoes
½ cup minced red onion
½ cup shredded Parmesan
  cheese (optional)

This is my go-to breakfast when we're headed out on a road trip. I prepare it the night before, pop it in the oven for 15 minutes while we get dressed and put our bags in the car, and then put the cooked muffins in a cloth lunch sack to take with us. They're especially helpful on long trips because gluten-free food is difficult to find at roadside restaurants.

1. Preheat the oven to 350°F.

2. Line a 12-cup muffin tin with paper liners.

3. In a large liquid measuring cup or juice pitcher, whisk the eggs and salt thoroughly.

4. Evenly divide the spinach, tomatoes, and onion among the 12 muffin cups.

5. Sprinkle each with an equal amount of Parmesan cheese (if using).

6. Pour the egg mixture evenly among the muffin cups to fill. Bake for 15 minutes or until set.

7. Cool for 5 minutes before serving.

COOKING TIP Parchment paper liners tend to release the muffin cups better than traditional paper liners. However, you can also brush the liners with oil or spray them with gluten-free cooking spray so they release easily.

PER SERVING Calories 143; Total Carbohydrates 3g; Sugar 1g; Total Fat 10g; Saturated Fat 3g; Sodium 302mg; Protein 11g; Fiber 0g

SAUSAGE-EGG
Muffin Cups

SERVES 6 • PREP TIME: 5 MINUTES • COOK TIME: 15 MINUTES

DAIRY-FREE
NUT-FREE

12 eggs
½ teaspoon sea salt
12 ounces cooked, crumbled gluten-free sausage
½ cup minced red onion
¼ cup minced fresh basil (optional)

My husband prefers the Sun-Dried Tomato and Egg Muffin Cups (page 40), but this version is the kids' and my favorite. I typically leave the basil out of theirs and mince the onion finely. These are delicious with crumbled Italian sausage or a precooked chicken sausage—just read the label to ensure they do not contain gluten.

1. Preheat the oven to 350°F.

2. Line a 12-cup muffin tin with paper liners.

3. In a large liquid measuring cup or juice pitcher, whisk the eggs and salt thoroughly.

4. Evenly divide the sausage and onion among the 12 muffin cups.

5. Sprinkle with the basil (if using).

6. Pour the egg mixture evenly among the muffin cups to fill. Bake for 15 minutes or until set.

7. Cool for 5 minutes before serving.

INGREDIENT TIP When shopping for sausage, choose natural varieties without added sugar or nitrites/nitrates.

PER SERVING Calories 322; Total Carbohydrates 2g; Sugar 1g; Total Fat 25g; Saturated Fat 8g; Sodium 704mg; Protein 22g; Fiber 0g

PERFECT HASH BROWNS

SERVES 4 ° PREP TIME: 5 MINUTES ° COOK TIME: 10 MINUTES

ALLERGEN-FREE
NUT-FREE
ONE POT
VEGAN

2 large Russet potatoes,
  unpeeled, scrubbed
2 tablespoons canola oil
Sea salt
Freshly ground
  black pepper

Prepared hash browns sold in the frozen section of the grocery store are often lightly coated in flour and deep-fried in oil in which other foods coated in flour were cooked. Either way, they likely contain gluten (not to mention a lot of soybean oil). Make your own, much healthier, version in just minutes at home.

1. With a box grater or food processor, grate the potatoes. Working with a handful of potatoes at a time, wring out the excess moisture.

2. Heat a large skillet or sauté pan over medium-high heat. When the skillet is very hot, add the canola oil and tilt the pan to coat thoroughly. Allow the oil to heat for about 30 seconds, but do not let it smoke.

3. Sprinkle the potatoes over the entire surface of the hot pan and season with salt and pepper. Cook the potatoes, undisturbed, for 5 to 7 minutes to develop a deep golden-brown crust on the bottom. If the bottom is cooking too quickly, lower the heat to medium.

4. Use a metal spatula to flip the hash browns. Cook the other side for 3 to 5 minutes until golden brown and cooked through. Serve immediately.

COOKING TIP Preheat the pan before adding the oil. This prevents the potatoes from sticking. A nonstick skillet could also accomplish this, but it will not produce this crisp golden-brown exterior. A well-seasoned cast-iron skillet is another good tool for making hash browns.

PER SERVING Calories 135; Total Carbohydrates 17g; Sugar 1g; Total Fat 7g; Saturated Fat 1g; Sodium 65mg; Protein 2g; Fiber 3g

VEGETABLE SKILLET HASH
with Eggs

SERVES 4 ∘ PREP TIME: 1O MINUTES ∘ COOK TIME: 2O MINUTES

DAIRY-FREE
NUT-FREE
ONE POT
VEGETARIAN
MAKE ALLERGEN-FREE
MAKE VEGAN

2 tablespoons canola
  oil, divided
2 small sweet potatoes,
  peeled and diced
1 small zucchini, diced
1 red bell pepper, cored
  and thinly sliced
½ red onion, thinly sliced
Sea salt
Freshly ground pepper
1 tablespoon roughly
  chopped fresh parsley
1 tablespoon roughly
  chopped fresh basil
4 eggs

I just adore vegetables, so whenever I can sneak them into another meal or snack, I'm happy. Normal breakfast hashes are made with potatoes and sausage. This one gets a healthy upgrade with sweet potatoes, zucchini, and bell peppers. If you don't have fresh herbs, just skip them.

1. Heat a large skillet or sauté pan over medium-high heat until hot. Add 1 tablespoon of the canola oil and tilt the pan to coat.

2. Add the sweet potatoes and cook for 5 minutes.

3. Push the sweet potatoes to the side of the pan and add the zucchini. Sauté for 2 to 3 minutes.

4. Push the zucchini to the side of the pan and add the bell pepper and onion. Sauté for 2 to 3 minutes.

5. Stir everything together, season with salt and pepper, and continue cooking until the sweet potatoes are soft, about 5 minutes more. Transfer the vegetables to a serving dish and sprinkle with the parsley and basil.

6. Add the remaining 1 tablespoon canola oil to the pan and cook the eggs sunny-side up, or to your liking. Serve the eggs over the hash.

SUBSTITUTION TIP For an allergen-free and vegan dish, omit the eggs and enjoy this very veggie hash "neat."

PER SERVING Calories 236; Total Carbohydrates 26g; Sugar 3g; Total Fat 12g; Saturated Fat 2g; Sodium 134mg; Protein 8g; Fiber 5g

FLUFFY BISCUITS
and Sausage Gravy

SERVES 8 ° PREP TIME: 10 MINUTES ° COOK TIME: 15 MINUTES

EGG-FREE
NUT-FREE
MAKE DAIRY-FREE

FOR THE BISCUITS
1 ¾ cups Whole-Grain
  Gluten-Free Flour Blend
  (page 25), plus more for
  dusting and dipping
1 tablespoon aluminum-
  free, double-acting
  baking powder
½ teaspoon sea salt
4 tablespoons cold butter,
  cut into small pieces
½ cup milk

FOR THE GRAVY
8 ounces gluten-free
  pork sausage
3 tablespoons Whole-
  Grain Gluten-Free Flour
  Blend (page 25)
1 ½ cups whole milk
Sea salt
Freshly ground
  black pepper

I love biscuits and gravy so much, I enjoy them for dinner as well as breakfast! They're usually made with wheat flour, both the biscuits and the gravy, but this version will safely satisfy your cravings for fluffy biscuits without gluten.

TO MAKE THE BISCUITS

1. Preheat the oven to 450°F.

2. In a food processor, combine the flour blend, baking powder, and salt and pulse once or twice to integrate.

3. Add the butter and pulse a few times. You should still be able to see several tiny pieces of butter.

4. Pour in the milk and blend just until integrated.

5. Lightly dust a clean work surface with the flour blend and place the dough on it. With a rolling pin, roll out the dough to about a 1-inch thickness. Use a glass lightly dipped in the flour blend to cut out individual biscuits.

6. Roll out the scraps again to use the remaining dough. Transfer the biscuits to a baking sheet, and bake for 12 to 14 minutes, until puffy and golden brown.

TO MAKE THE GRAVY

1. While the biscuits are baking, in a large skillet or sauté pan over medium heat, cook the sausage for about 5 minutes, breaking it up with the back of a spoon, until browned and cooked through. Use a slotted spoon to transfer the sausage to a separate dish, leaving the drippings in the skillet.

2. Whisk the flour blend into the drippings, and cook for 1 to 2 minutes until bubbling.

3. Pour in the milk and whisk vigorously to break up the flour lumps. Bring to a simmer and cook for 2 to 3 minutes, stirring constantly, until thickened.

4. Stir the sausage into the gravy, and season with salt and pepper.

5. To serve, slice the biscuits in half and top with the sausage gravy.

SUBSTITUTION TIP To make this dairy-free, choose a nondairy milk with a high fat content, such as coconut milk.

PER SERVING Calories 299; Total Carbohydrates 28g; Sugar 3g; Total Fat 16g; Saturated Fat 7g; Sodium 397mg; Protein 11g; Fiber 1g

BLUEBERRY MUFFINS

MAKES 12 MUFFINS ∘ PREP TIME: 10 MINUTES ∘ COOK TIME: 15 TO 18 MINUTES

NUT-FREE
VEGETARIAN
MAKE DAIRY-FREE

2 cups Whole-Grain
  Gluten-Free Flour
  Blend (page 25)
1 tablespoon aluminum-
  free, double-acting
  baking powder
½ teaspoon sea salt
2 eggs
¾ cup milk
½ cup sugar
⅓ cup canola oil
1 teaspoon vanilla extract
½ teaspoon finely grated
  fresh lemon zest
1 cup fresh or frozen
  blueberries

I prefer making blueberry muffins with frozen blue-berries because they bleed a beautiful purple color into the batter. But, if it's blueberry season where you live, use fresh ones. They will hold up better in baking and keep the batter a creamy white color.

1. Preheat the oven to 375°F.

2. Line a 12-cup muffin tin with paper liners.

3. In a large bowl, mix the flour blend, baking powder, and salt.

4. In a medium bowl, whisk the eggs, milk, sugar, canola oil, vanilla, and lemon zest. Stir the milk mixture into the flour mixture until just combined.

5. Fold in the blueberries.

6. Evenly divide the batter among the muffin cups. Bake for 15 to 18 minutes until golden brown and puffy.

7. Cool for 5 minutes before removing from the muffin tin.

SUBSTITUTION TIP To make this dairy-free, use a nondairy milk, such as unsweetened almond or soy milk. For a fun variation, use orange zest instead of lemon zest and cranberries in place of the blueberries.

PER SERVING Calories 187; Total Carbohydrates 27g; Sugar 10g; Total Fat 7g; Saturated Fat 1g; Sodium 97mg; Protein 4g; Fiber 1g

MORNING GLORY MUFFINS

MAKES 12 MUFFINS ○ PREP TIME: 10 MINUTES ○ COOK TIME: 15 TO 18 MINUTES

DAIRY-FREE
VEGETARIAN
MAKE NUT-FREE

1 ½ cups Whole-Grain
  Gluten-Free Flour
  Blend (page 25)
1 teaspoon baking soda
1 teaspoon ground
  cinnamon
½ teaspoon freshly
  ground nutmeg
½ teaspoon sea salt
2 eggs
1 ripe banana, mashed
⅓ cup canola oil
¼ cup packed
  brown sugar
1 carrot, shredded
1 small apple, cored
  and diced
½ cup raisins
¼ cup finely chopped
  walnuts (optional)

I grew up on the wheat flour version of these muffins, but I actually prefer this gluten-free version. They're a hodgepodge of pantry staples I always seem to have on hand, so they come together easily without having to pick up any special groceries.

1. Preheat the oven to 375°F.

2. Line a 12-cup muffin tin with paper liners.

3. In a large bowl, mix together the flour blend, baking soda, cinnamon, nutmeg, and salt.

4. In a medium bowl, whisk the eggs, banana, canola oil, and brown sugar. Stir the egg mixture into the flour mixture until just combined.

5. Fold in the carrot, apple, raisins, and walnuts (if using).

6. Evenly divide the batter among the muffin cups. Bake for 15 to 18 minutes, until golden brown and puffy.

7. Cool for 5 minutes before removing from the muffin tin.

SUBSTITUTION TIP Use shredded zucchini in place of the carrot if that's what you have on hand.

PER SERVING Calories 170; Total Carbohydrates 25g; Sugar 10g; Total Fat 7g; Saturated Fat 1g; Sodium 198mg; Protein 3g; Fiber 2g

COFFEE CAKE

SERVES 9 ° PREP TIME: 5 MINUTES ° COOK TIME: 25 MINUTES

NUT-FREE
VEGETARIAN
MAKE DAIRY-FREE

6 tablespoons melted
butter, divided, plus more
for coating the dish
2 cups Whole-Grain
Gluten-Free Flour Blend
(page 25), divided
¾ cup packed brown
sugar, divided
2½ teaspoons aluminum-
free, double-acting
baking powder
½ teaspoon plus pinch
sea salt, divided
2 teaspoons ground
cinnamon, divided
1 egg
½ cup milk
1 teaspoon vanilla extract

I'm not going to argue that this is a healthy break-fast recipe, but some days (hint: Saturdays) warrant a breakfast filled with all the healthy menu options—eggs, plain yogurt, and fruit—*and* a special treat. This is perfect for leisurely brunches and to be enjoyed, as its name suggests, with no more than a cup of coffee.

1. Preheat the oven to 350°F.

2. Coat the inside of an 8-by-8-inch baking dish with butter and set aside.

3. In a large bowl, combine 1½ cups of the flour blend, ½ cup of the brown sugar, the baking powder, ½ teaspoon of the salt, and 1 teaspoon of the cinnamon. Whisk to combine. Make a well in the center of the ingredients.

4. Into the well, add the egg, milk, 2 tablespoons of the melted butter, and the vanilla. Whisk just until blended. Pour the cake batter into the prepared pan.

5. In a medium bowl, combine the remaining ½ cup flour blend, ¼ cup brown sugar, pinch salt, 1 teaspoon cinnamon, and 4 tablespoons melted butter. Use your hands to combine the mixture until it resembles coarse crumbs. Sprinkle over the cake.

6. Bake for 25 minutes, or until a cake tester inserted into the center of the cake comes out clean.

7. Cool completely before slicing and serving.

SERVING TIP Feeling fancy? Make a cinnamon swirl cake. Whisk 1 tablespoon cinnamon with 1 tablespoon sugar and 2 tablespoons water. Drizzle over the cake and swirl with a toothpick before topping with the crumb layer.

SUBSTITUTION TIP To make this dairy-free, use nondairy milk in place of the milk and canola oil in place of the butter.

PER SERVING Calories 233; Total Carbohydrates 35g; Sugar 13g; Total Fat 9g; Saturated Fat 5g; Sodium 178mg; Protein 4g; Fiber 1g

CLASSIC SCONES

MAKES 8 SCONES ∘ PREP TIME: 5 MINUTES ∘ COOK TIME: 15 MINUTES

NUT-FREE
VEGETARIAN
MAKE DAIRY-FREE

1¾ cups Whole-Grain Gluten-Free Flour Blend (page 25), plus more for dusting
2½ teaspoons aluminum-free, double-acting baking powder
¼ cup sugar
½ teaspoon sea salt
4 tablespoons cold butter, cut into pieces
2 eggs
⅓ cup heavy (whipping) cream
¼ teaspoon vanilla extract

I lived in England for the better part of a year, but sadly, never enjoyed scones because I couldn't find any that were gluten-free. It's about five years late, but it's time to have my scones and eat them too! Jazz things up by folding in currants, dried cranberries, and orange zest, or even white chocolate chips and a handful of fresh raspberries.

1. Preheat the oven to 425°F.

2. In a food processor, combine the flour blend, baking powder, sugar, and salt. Pulse 1 to 2 times, just to integrate.

3. Add the butter and pulse until the mixture resembles coarse sand.

4. Add the eggs, heavy cream, and vanilla, and blend for a few seconds, just until integrated.

5. On a lightly floured work surface, roll out the dough to a 1-inch-thick round. Cut into 8 wedges and place on a baking sheet.

6. Bake for 15 minutes until lightly browned.

SUBSTITUTION TIP For dairy-free scones, use shortening, and replace the heavy cream with coconut cream. It can be purchased from Trader Joe's, or refrigerate a can of full-fat coconut milk overnight and carefully scoop off the top layer of cream.

PER SERVING Calories 209; Total Carbohydrates 28g; Sugar 6g; Total Fat 9g; Saturated Fat 5g; Sodium 177mg; Protein 4g; Fiber 1g

CHEDDAR-JALAPEÑO SCONES

MAKES 8 SCONES ∘ PREP TIME: 5 MINUTES ∘ COOK TIME: 15 MINUTES

NUT-FREE
VEGETARIAN

1 ¾ cups Whole-Grain
  Gluten-Free Flour Blend
  (page 25), plus more
  for dusting
2 ½ teaspoons aluminum-
  free, double-acting
  baking powder
½ teaspoon sea salt
4 tablespoons cold butter,
  cut into pieces
2 eggs
⅓ cup heavy
  (whipping) cream
1 cup shredded sharp
  Cheddar cheese
¼ cup canned jalapeño
  peppers, drained
  and minced

These scones are delicious topped with scrambled eggs, or enjoyed on their own on your way out the door to work. They also work as a tasty side dish in school lunches. Adjust the amount of jalapeño based on your desired level of spiciness.

1. Preheat the oven to 425°F.

2. In a food processor, combine the flour blend, baking powder, and salt. Pulse 1 to 2 times, just to integrate.

3. Add the butter and pulse until the mixture resembles coarse sand.

4. Add the eggs and heavy cream, and blend for a few seconds, just until integrated.

5. Fold in the Cheddar cheese and jalapeños.

6. Roll out the dough on a lightly floured work surface to a 1-inch-thick round. Cut into 8 wedges and place on a baking sheet.

7. Bake for 15 minutes until lightly browned.

SUBSTITUTION TIP To use fresh peppers, stem and core 1 fresh jalapeño pepper, mince it, and fold it into the batter.

PER SERVING Calories 243; Total Carbohydrates 22g; Sugar 0g; Total Fat 14g; Saturated Fat 8g; Sodium 319mg; Protein 8g; Fiber 1g

LEMON CRÊPES

MAKES 8 CRÊPES ° PREP TIME: 5 MINUTES ° COOK TIME: 10 MINUTES

NUT-FREE
VEGETARIAN
MAKE DAIRY-FREE

4 eggs
¼ cup tapioca
  flour (starch)
¼ cup milk
1 teaspoon finely grated
  fresh lemon zest
Pinch sea salt
4 tablespoons
  butter, divided

When my husband and I were dating in college, we often met at a quirky coffee shop in Northwest Portland to study. The shop also served crêpes, which they spread onto specialized griddles with a squeegee-like tool for the thinnest, most delicate crêpes imaginable. This is the closest recipe I have found for these authentically French pancakes.

1. In a blender, process the eggs, tapioca flour, milk, lemon zest, and salt until blended. Let rest briefly while you heat the pan.

2. Heat an 8-inch skillet or sauté pan over medium heat. Melt 1 to 2 teaspoons of the butter in the pan.

3. Pour a scant ¼ cup of crêpe batter into the pan, tilting the pan to coat the bottom. Cook until nearly set.

4. Carefully slide a spatula under the crêpe and flip to cook the other side. Transfer to a warmed plate.

5. Repeat with the remaining batter, stacking the finished crêpes on the plate.

SERVING TIP To make a crêpe cake, double this recipe, cook the crêpes as directed, and then spread a thin layer of jam, lemon curd, Nutella, or other sweet filling between the crêpes. Stack and shower with powdered sugar.

COOKING TIP I do not cook with nonstick cookware, but it certainly makes cooking crêpes easier, and you can use less butter.

SUBSTITUTION TIP To make this dairy-free, use an unsweetened, nondairy milk such as almond or soy milk.

PER SERVING Calories 103; Total Carbohydrates 5g; Sugar 1g; Total Fat 8g; Saturated Fat 4g; Sodium 107mg; Protein 3g; Fiber 0g

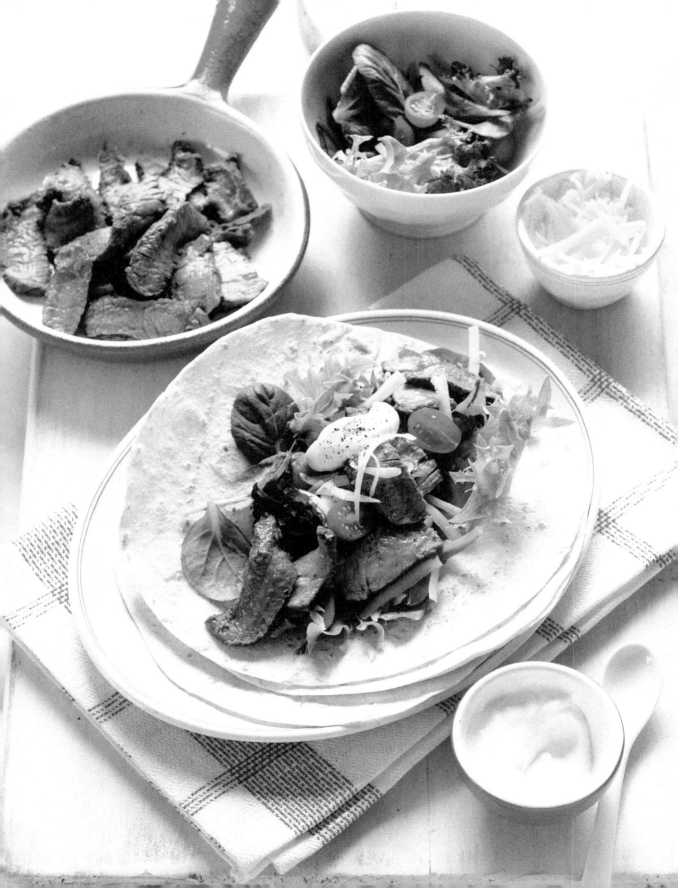

CHAPTER Three

LUNCH

HUMMUS RICE CAKES

SERVES 4 ∘ PREP TIME: 5 MINUTES

ALLERGEN-FREE
NUT-FREE
VEGAN

8 gluten-free brown
  rice cakes
1½ cups prepared
  hummus, divided
1 cucumber, thinly sliced
½ red onion, thinly sliced
4 vine-ripened tomatoes,
  thinly sliced
Freshly ground
  black pepper

This recipe requires no actual cooking or even much preparation. Simply gather the ingredients, pack them into lunch sacks, and look forward to a healthy, filling lunch.

1. Slather each rice cake with about 3 tablespoons of hummus.

2. Top each with cucumber, onion, and tomato. Season with pepper.

SERVING TIP For more protein, serve with a few crumbles of feta cheese.

PER SERVING Calories 315; Total Carbohydrates 50g; Sugar 5g; Total Fat 10g; Saturated Fat 1g; Sodium 433mg; Protein 11g; Fiber 10g

ALMOND BUTTER AND BANANA
Rice Cakes

SERVES 4 ∘ PREP TIME: 5 MINUTES

VEGAN

8 gluten-free
  brown rice cakes
1 cup almond
  butter, divided
2 bananas, sliced
¼ teaspoon ground
  cinnamon

This is one of my boys' favorite lunches. In fact, Cole begged to take a picture of it when I made it last time. Think of it as an open-faced sandwich—the toppings can include a variety of items, but you really can't go wrong with bananas and cinnamon. Cole's favorite version of this lunch is with a couple dark chocolate chips and a few raisins.

1. Slather each rice cake with about 2 tablespoons of almond butter.

2. Top with bananas and a light dusting of cinnamon.

SERVING TIP If you're sending this in a school lunch box, wrap each rice cake in plastic wrap before packing.

PER SERVING Calories 510; Total Carbohydrates 39g; Sugar 6g; Total Fat 38g; Saturated Fat 4g; Sodium 6mg; Protein 1g; Fiber 4g

CHICKEN SALAD WITH
Apples and Mint

SERVES 2 ∘ PREP TIME: 5 MINUTES

DAIRY-FREE
NUT-FREE
MAKE ALLERGEN-FREE
MAKE EGG-FREE

2 cups diced cooked
  chicken breast
2 tablespoons minced
  fresh mint
1 shallot, minced
1 Pink Lady apple or
  another sweet-tart
  variety, cored
  and julienned
1 tablespoon freshly
  squeezed lemon juice
2 tablespoons mayonnaise
Freshly ground
  black pepper

I like to make this chicken salad using leftover meat from the Basic Roast Chicken (page 128). It is perfect as a relatively low-carb lunch on its own. Or wrap it in a gluten-free tortilla and add a handful of mixed greens. Keep it properly chilled so the mayonnaise does not spoil.

1. In a medium bowl, mix the chicken, mint, shallot, and apple.

2. Add the lemon juice and mayonnaise, and stir to coat all ingredients with the dressing.

3. Season with pepper.

SUBSTITUTION TIP For an allergen-free and egg-free recipe, use a vegan mayonnaise without soybean oil.

PER SERVING Calories 299; Total Carbohydrates 18g; Sugar 11g; Total Fat 9g; Saturated Fat 1g; Sodium 240mg; Protein 37g; Fiber 3g

CURRIED CHICKEN SALAD

SERVES 2 ° PREP TIME: 10 MINUTES

2 cups diced cooked
  chicken breast
1 celery stalk, diced
½ cup halved
  green grapes
¼ cup finely diced
  red onion
¼ cup roughly chopped
  roasted cashews
2 tablespoons mayonnaise
1 tablespoon freshly
  squeezed lime juice
1 teaspoon gluten-free
  curry powder
1 teaspoon minced peeled
  fresh ginger
1 teaspoon minced garlic
Freshly ground
  black pepper

I love the combination of sweet grapes, pungent curry powder, and spicy onion and garlic in this flavorful chicken salad. Wrap it in butter lettuce leaves for a low-carb option or in a gluten-free tortilla with a handful of fresh arugula for a more filling lunch.

1. In a medium bowl, mix the chicken, celery, grapes, onion, and cashews.

2. In a small bowl, whisk the mayonnaise, lime juice, curry powder, ginger, and garlic.

3. Pour the dressing over the chicken mixture and stir to coat thoroughly.

4. Season with pepper.

SUBSTITUTION TIP I like to grate ginger and garlic using a Microplane grater for the finest texture. The tool yields almost a purée consistency that disburses readily throughout the salad.

PER SERVING Calories 373; Total Carbohydrates 16g; Sugar 6g; Total Fat 17g; Saturated Fat 2g; Sodium 247mg; Protein 40g; Fiber 2g

GREEK SALAD

SERVES 4 ∘ PREP TIME: 10 MINUTES

EGG-FREE
NUT-FREE
VEGETARIAN
MAKE ALLERGEN-FREE
MAKE DAIRY-FREE

½ cup extra-virgin olive oil
¼ cup red wine vinegar
1 teaspoon fresh
    thyme leaves
1 teaspoon fresh minced
    oregano leaves
1 small garlic
    clove, minced
Sea salt
Freshly ground
    black pepper
1 head romaine lettuce,
    rinsed, dried, and roughly
    chopped (about 10 cups)
1 English cucumber, diced
1 pint grape tomatoes
½ red onion, thinly sliced
1 cup pitted
    Kalamata olives
1 cup crumbled
    feta cheese

The bold flavors of Kalamata olives, red wine vinegar, and feta cheese in this salad will keep you watching the clock all morning for lunchtime to roll around. If you cannot eat cow's milk dairy, look for a sheep's milk feta. To make this salad a filling dinner, add 1 pound of cooked and chilled seafood, such as shrimp, scallops, or calamari.

1. In a small sealable jar, combine the olive oil, vinegar, thyme, oregano, and garlic. Season with salt and pepper. Seal the lid and shake to emulsify the ingredients.

2. In a large salad bowl, mix the romaine lettuce, cucumber, tomatoes, onion, and olives. Add the dressing and toss to coat thoroughly.

3. Top with the feta cheese and serve.

SERVING TIP To pack this in a lunch box, divide the salad among large sealable containers. Store the dressing and feta cheese in separate sealed jars or plastic containers.

SUBSTITUTION TIP To make this allergen-free and dairy-free, omit the feta cheese.

PER SERVING Calories 412; Total Carbohydrates 16g; Sugar 7g; Total Fat 37g; Saturated Fat 10g; Sodium 785mg; Protein 8g; Fiber 4g

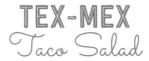

TEX-MEX
Taco Salad

SERVES 4 ∘ PREP TIME: 5 MINUTES

EGG-FREE
NUT-FREE
VEGETARIAN
MAKE DAIRY-FREE
MAKE VEGAN

1 (15-ounce) can black beans, drained but not rinsed

1 tablespoon Taco Seasoning (page 216), or purchased gluten-free taco seasoning

1 tablespoon freshly squeezed lime juice

1 tablespoon ketchup

1 head romaine lettuce, roughly chopped

1 cup frozen roasted corn kernels, thawed

2 avocados, diced

1 cup pico de gallo salsa

1 cup shredded Cheddar cheese

4 cups corn chips

I often make this recipe with ground beef, but the canned black beans are already cooked and provide a convenient lunch option for busy mornings. Either one tastes great! Store all ingredients in separate containers or in a bento-style lunch box.

1. In a medium bowl, thoroughly mix the black beans, taco seasoning, lime juice, and ketchup. Set aside.

2. Evenly divide the romaine lettuce among 4 serving dishes. Top each with equal amounts of the seasoned black beans, corn, avocado, pico de gallo, and Cheddar cheese. Serve the corn chips on the side.

SUBSTITUTION TIP Skip the cheese to make this recipe dairy-free and vegan.

PER SERVING Calories 728; Total Carbohydrates 79g; Sugar 8g; Total Fat 38g; Saturated Fat 11g; Sodium 797mg; Protein 26g; Fiber 20g

MIXED GREENS WITH
Chicken, Mango, and Cashews

SERVES 4 ∘ PREP TIME: 10 MINUTES

DAIRY-FREE
EGG-FREE
MAKE NUT-FREE

⅓ cup canola oil
2 tablespoons gluten-free
  soy sauce
2 tablespoons freshly
  squeezed lime juice
1 tablespoon sesame oil
1 garlic clove, minced
Pinch red pepper flakes
6 cups roughly chopped
  mixed green lettuces
2 cups shredded cabbage
½ cup roughly chopped
  fresh cilantro
¼ cup roughly chopped
  fresh mint leaves
3 cups chopped cooked
  chicken breast
1 cup diced mango
  (from 1 whole fruit)
½ cup roughly chopped
  toasted cashews
  (optional)

The sweet mango, tangy dressing, and salty cashews make this everyday lunch anything but average. For a nut-free meal, omit the cashews or replace them with toasted sesame seeds. I like to make one batch of the dressing and enjoy it a couple times throughout the week. If you plan to pack this for lunches, divide the salad among large sealable containers, keeping the dressing in a separate sealable jar.

1. In a sealable jar, combine the canola oil, soy sauce, lime juice, sesame oil, garlic, and red pepper flakes. Seal the lid and shake to emulsify the ingredients.

2. In a large salad bowl, mix the lettuces, cabbage, cilantro, and mint.

3. Just before serving, add the dressing and toss the salad to coat.

4. Top with the chicken and mango, and finish with the toasted cashews (if using).

COOKING TIP To save time, purchase precooked chicken (be sure it's gluten-free) or cook several chicken breasts at once, cool completely, slice, and freeze in individual serving sizes. For even more time savings, look for diced fresh mango refrigerated in the produce section of your local grocery.

PER SERVING Calories 393; Total Carbohydrates 15g; Sugar 10g; Total Fat 25g; Saturated Fat 2g; Sodium 564mg; Protein 29g; Fiber 3g

KALE SALAD WITH
Chicken and Avocado

SERVES 2 ∘ PREP TIME: 15 MINUTES

1 bunch fresh kale, any variety, thoroughly washed and dried, ribs removed, and roughly chopped

Sea salt

2 tablespoons extra-virgin olive oil

1 teaspoon freshly squeezed lemon juice

1 teaspoon red wine vinegar

2 cups chopped cooked skinless chicken breast

1 avocado, diced

2 tablespoons roughly chopped toasted hazelnuts (optional)

I know the kale craze is mostly over, but true love lasts a lifetime. I still make this scrumptious kale salad for lunch at least once a week. If avocados are not in season, add some grape tomatoes instead.

1. Put the kale into a large salad bowl and season with salt.

2. Drizzle the olive oil over the kale and massage it with your hands until the kale begins to feel soft and release some of its liquid, about 15 seconds.

3. Sprinkle with the lemon juice and vinegar, and toss to coat.

4. Divide the salad between 2 serving plates and top with the chicken breast and diced avocado.

5. Finish with the hazelnuts (if using).

SERVING TIP If you're preparing this salad to take to work, double the amount of dressing ingredients and store in a sealable jar apart from the remaining salad ingredients.

PER SERVING Calories 611; Total Carbohydrates 30g; Sugar 1g; Total Fat 38g; Saturated Fat 6g; Sodium 341mg; Protein 44g; Fiber 10g

FARMERS' MARKET
Kale Salad

SERVES 2 ∘ PREP TIME: 10 MINUTES

1 bunch fresh kale, any variety, thoroughly washed and dried, ribs removed, and roughly chopped

2 cups chickpeas, rinsed and drained

1 cup grape tomatoes

1 cup diced zucchini

½ red onion, thinly sliced

¼ cup extra-virgin olive oil

1 tablespoon freshly squeezed lemon juice

1 tablespoon red wine vinegar

1 garlic clove, minced

Sea salt

Freshly ground black pepper

This vegetable salad is filling and delicious and makes the perfect entrée. You can use whatever vegetables are fresh and in season where you live.

1. In a large salad bowl, mix the kale, chickpeas, tomatoes, zucchini, and onion.

2. In a sealable jar, combine the olive oil, lemon juice, vinegar, and garlic. Season with salt and pepper. Seal the lid and shake the jar to emulsify the ingredients.

3. Just before serving, pour the dressing over the salad and gently toss to mix.

INGREDIENT TIP Roasted vegetables are especially good in this salad. If you're cooking vegetables for dinner, roast the tomatoes, zucchini, and onion and then refrigerate to enjoy for lunch the next day.

PER SERVING Calories 687; Total Carbohydrates 92g; Sugar 16g; Total Fat 32g; Saturated Fat 4g; Sodium 245mg; Protein 28g; Fiber 23g

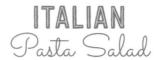

ITALIAN
Pasta Salad

SERVES 4 ∘ PREP TIME: 5 MINUTES ∘ COOK TIME: 10 MINUTES

NUT-FREE
VEGAN

8 ounces gluten-free
  penne pasta or
  elbow pasta
¼ cup extra-virgin olive oil
2 tablespoons red
  wine vinegar
1 garlic clove, minced
1 teaspoon minced
  fresh oregano
Sea salt
Freshly ground
  black pepper
½ cup oil-packed sun-
  dried tomatoes, drained
  and cut into thin strips
1 (12-ounce) jar roasted
  red peppers, drained and
  roughly chopped
2 cups fresh baby spinach,
  washed, dried, and
  roughly chopped
¼ cup roughly chopped
  fresh flat-leaf parsley

Sun-dried tomatoes pack a huge flavor punch in such a small package. I wrote a cookbook on healthy dehydrating and I prefer to dry my own tomatoes to use in this recipe, but the jarred varieties are equally stellar. Choose one with a delicious herb marinade for even more flavor.

1. Bring a large pot of salted water to a boil over high heat. Cook the pasta according to the package directions. Drain thoroughly and transfer to a large bowl.

2. Meanwhile, in a liquid measuring cup, combine the olive oil, vinegar, garlic, and oregano. Season with salt and pepper. Whisk to emulsify the ingredients.

3. Pour the dressing over the warm pasta.

4. Add the tomatoes, red peppers, spinach, and parsley. Gently toss to mix. The residual heat from the pasta will wilt the spinach slightly.

5. Evenly divide the salad among 4 serving bowls, or transfer to individual sealable containers and refrigerate until ready to serve.

INGREDIENT TIP Can't imagine a meal without meat? Add 4 ounces of sliced salami or another cured meat to this salad. It is also great with sliced grilled chicken.

PER SERVING Calories 289; Total Carbohydrates 34g; Sugar 1g; Total Fat 14g; Saturated Fat 2g; Sodium 90mg; Protein 8g; Fiber 1g

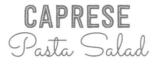

CAPRESE
Pasta Salad

SERVES 4 ° PREP TIME: 5 MINUTES ° COOK TIME: 10 MINUTES

EGG-FREE
NUT-FREE
SPLURGE-WORTHY
VEGETARIAN

8 ounces gluten-free
  penne pasta or
  elbow pasta
¼ cup extra-virgin olive oil
2 tablespoons balsamic
  vinegar
Sea salt
Freshly ground
  black pepper
1 pint grape tomatoes
8 ounces baby
  bocconcini, drained
1 cup roughly chopped
  fresh basil

Baby bocconcini are small balls of fresh mozzarella cheese, and they're just about the cutest culinary creation. They work perfectly in this vegetarian salad inspired by caprese salad, which is a stack of sliced fresh mozzarella, tomatoes, and fresh basil drizzled with olive oil and balsamic vinegar.

1. Bring a large pot of salted water to a boil over high heat. Cook the pasta according to the package directions. Drain, rinse under cold water, drain again thoroughly, and transfer to a large bowl.

2. Pour the olive oil and vinegar over the pasta. Season with salt and pepper, and gently toss to mix.

3. Add the tomatoes, bocconcini, and basil. Gently toss again to mix.

4. Evenly divide the salad among 4 serving bowls, or transfer to individual sealable containers and refrigerate until ready to serve.

INGREDIENT TIP If you can't find bocconcini, cut a larger fresh mozzarella ball into cubes. Alternatively, use traditional mozzarella cheese, cut into cubes, and store separately from the salad until ready to serve.

PER SERVING Calories 493; Total Carbohydrates 39g; Sugar 2g; Total Fat 28g; Saturated Fat 12g; Sodium 443mg; Protein 22g; Fiber 1g

CARNE ASADA BOWLS

SERVES 2 ∘ PREP TIME: 10 MINUTES ∘ COOK TIME: 10 MINUTES

ALLERGEN-FREE
DAIRY-FREE
EGG-FREE
NUT-FREE

1 tablespoon freshly
  squeezed lime juice
1 tablespoon extra-virgin
  olive oil
1 teaspoon minced garlic
1 teaspoon ground cumin
1 teaspoon minced
  fresh oregano
1 teaspoon ancho
  chile powder
¼ teaspoon sea salt
Freshly ground
  black pepper
8 ounces flank steak
2 cups cooked brown rice
¼ cup minced red onion
1 cup roasted
  tomato salsa
½ cup prepared
  guacamole
1 lime, cut into 4 wedges

I enjoy this salad bowl both freshly cooked and hot, or made ahead of time and chilled. Its full, rich flavor makes it a regular favorite.

1. In a shallow dish large enough to hold the steak, whisk the lime juice, olive oil, garlic, cumin, oregano, ancho chile powder, and salt. Season with pepper.

2. Coat the flank steak in the mixture and let rest for 5 minutes.

3. Meanwhile, preheat a grill pan over medium-high heat until very hot, about 5 minutes.

4. Sear the flank steak for 3 to 5 minutes on each side for medium-rare. Remove to a cutting board and let rest for 5 minutes before thinly slicing.

5. In the same grill pan, heat the brown rice and divide between 2 serving dishes.

6. Top each with the sliced steak, onion, salsa, and guacamole.

7. Serve with the lime wedges.

VARIATION TIP Skip the rice and serve this as a salad tucked into some gluten-free tortillas. Combine some mixed lettuces, fresh spinach, and grape tomatoes. Sprinkle with lime juice and divide among the tortillas. Top with steak slices, a sprinkle of shredded mozzarella cheese, and a dollop of sour cream. Of course, this won't be dairy-free, but it's still delicious and gluten-free.

PER SERVING Calories 715; Total Carbohydrates 85g; Sugar 5g; Total Fat 24g; Saturated Fat 6g; Sodium 1139mg; Protein 42g; Fiber 7g

THREE SISTERS BLISS BOWLS
with Cashew Aioli

SERVES 4 ° PREP TIME: 10 MINUTES ° COOK TIME: 10 MINUTES

VEGAN

½ cup cashews

1 cup boiling water

2 cups cubed
butternut squash

1 garlic clove

1 tablespoon freshly
squeezed lemon juice

1 tablespoon extra-virgin
olive oil

Sea salt

Freshly ground pepper

1 (15-ounce) can pinto
beans, rinsed and
drained

2 cups frozen corn
kernels, thawed

2 cups shredded
fresh kale

¼ cup dried cranberries

¼ cup pepitas (shelled
pumpkin seeds)

Corn, beans, and winter squash comprise the famous Three Sisters, which were often raised as companion crops in many Native American cultures. Or, in other words, when planted together, the Three Sisters help each other grow. And they are delightful served together in this dish. The cashew aioli is tangy, delicious, and naturally vegan. If you don't feel like making it, drizzle the salad with tahini or another creamy dressing.

1. In a heatproof container, cover the cashews with the boiling water and set aside for 10 minutes to soak.

2. Put a steamer basket into a medium pot and add 1 inch water. Put the butternut squash into the steamer basket. Bring the water to a simmer over medium heat, cover, and cook for 10 minutes, or until the squash is tender.

3. Rinse and drain the cashews. Put them in a blender with the garlic, lemon juice, and olive oil. Purée until smooth, adding water as needed to get things moving. Season with salt and pepper.

4. Evenly divide the cooked squash among 4 serving bowls.

5. To each, add pinto beans, corn, and shredded kale.

6. Drizzle with the cashew aioli, and then top with dried cranberries and pepitas.

SERVING TIP If you're packing this for lunch, place the ingredients into a Mason jar in the order listed, beginning with the cashew aioli, followed by cooked butternut squash, beans, corn, kale, cranberries, and pepitas. To eat, turn the jar upside down and shake to coat with the dressing.

PER SERVING Calories 463; Total Carbohydrates 66g; Sugar 6g; Total Fat 17g; Saturated Fat 3g; Sodium 88mg; Protein 19g; Fiber 13g

BROWN RICE
Baja Bowls

SERVES 2 ∘ PREP TIME: 3 MINUTES ∘ COOK TIME: 2 MINUTES

NUT-FREE
ONE POT
VEGAN

2 cups cooked brown rice
1 cup frozen roasted
  corn kernels, thawed
1 cup pico de gallo salsa
1 cup prepared guacamole
¼ cup minced
  fresh cilantro
1 lime, cut into 4 wedges

This recipe can take 5 minutes if you purchase prepared ingredients or an hour if you want to cook the brown rice and make the salsa and guacamole from scratch. On busy workdays, I opt for the former option! It's a filling vegan lunch with protein, complex carbohydrates, and healthy fat.

1. In a skillet or sauté pan, heat the brown rice and roasted corn. Divide between 2 serving dishes.

2. Top each with the pico de gallo, guacamole, and cilantro and serve with lime wedges.

INGREDIENT TIP Some people have a certain genetic predisposition in which they taste an overwhelmingly soapy aroma and flavor in cilantro, which may also cause an allergic reaction. If you're among them, simply leave it out of this recipe.

PER SERVING Calories 524; Total Carbohydrates 100g; Sugar 7g; Total Fat 11g; Saturated Fat 2g; Sodium 957mg; Protein 12g; Fiber 9g

TURKEY-CRANBERRY
Lettuce Wraps

SERVES 2 ° PREP TIME: 5 MINUTES

EGG-FREE
NUT-FREE

2 ounces cream cheese, at room temperature, divided
2 gluten-free tortillas
¼ cup dried cranberries, divided
4 ounces gluten-free sliced turkey breast, divided
1 cup shredded romaine lettuce, divided

The flavors of Thanksgiving permeate this sweet and savory turkey wrap. For a low-carb option, use lettuce leaves instead of gluten-free tortillas.

1. Spread half of the cream cheese over each tortilla.

2. Top each with half of the cranberries, turkey, and lettuce, in that order.

3. Roll the tortillas, folding in each end. Wrap in plastic wrap or parchment paper and keep cold until ready to serve.

SERVING TIP These wraps will keep for a few hours, but store the ingredients separately if you intend to consume them more than 6 hours from the time of preparation.

PER SERVING Calories 221; Total Carbohydrates 16g; Sugar 3g; Total Fat 12g; Saturated Fat 7g; Sodium 672mg; Protein 13g; Fiber 3g

COLLARD GUACAMOLE
Veggie Wraps

SERVES 2 ° PREP TIME: 5 MINUTES

ALLERGEN-FREE
NUT-FREE
VEGAN

6 large collard leaves,
 thick ribs carefully
 removed
1 cup prepared
 guacamole, divided
1 red bell pepper, cored
 and thinly sliced
1 cucumber, cut
 into spears
2 carrots, shredded

The raw vegan movement has, at times, piqued my interest. While exploring raw recipes, I discovered the beauty of vegetable wraps, which are naturally gluten-free. However, if collard greens aren't your thing, use gluten-free spinach tortillas instead, and add a handful of shredded lettuce to the wrap.

1. Slather each collard leaf with a few tablespoons of the guacamole.

2. Top each with a few slices of bell pepper and cucumber.

3. Sprinkle with the shredded carrot, then roll each leaf into a tight cylinder. Serve immediately.

SERVING TIP For more protein, add a slice of chicken or tofu to each wrap.

SUBSTITUTION TIP You can also use prepared hummus in place of the guacamole.

PER SERVING Calories 162; Total Carbohydrates 22g; Sugar 9g; Total Fat 9g; Saturated Fat 1g; Sodium 226mg; Protein 4g; Fiber 7g

CHICKEN LETTUCE CUPS

SERVES 4 ∘ PREP TIME: 10 MINUTES ∘ COOK TIME: 8 MINUTES

DAIRY-FREE
EGG-FREE
MAKE NUT-FREE

1 tablespoon sesame oil

1 ½ pounds boneless skinless chicken thighs, finely diced

1 tablespoon peeled minced fresh ginger

1 tablespoon minced garlic

Pinch red pepper flakes

1 tablespoon gluten-free soy sauce

1 tablespoon freshly squeezed lime juice

Sea salt

Freshly ground black pepper

1 head butter lettuce, leaves separated

½ red onion, minced

¼ cup minced fresh cilantro

¼ cup roughly chopped peanuts (optional)

These are a favorite on Asian fusion restaurant menus and so easy to create at home and pack for lunch. Even the kids love them, though omit the red pepper flakes for a milder version. To make the recipe nut-free, omit the peanuts.

1. In a large skillet or sauté pan over medium-high heat, heat the sesame oil.

2. Add the chicken and sauté for 5 minutes.

3. Stir in the ginger, garlic, and red pepper flakes. Continue cooking for about 2 minutes more until the chicken is cooked through and gently browned.

4. Add the soy sauce and lime juice and cook for 30 seconds more. Season with salt and pepper.

5. Serve the chicken spooned into the lettuce leaves and garnished with onion, cilantro, and peanuts.

SERVING TIP Send this to work or school in a lunch box by packing the chicken with the minced onion, cilantro, and peanuts. Store the lettuce leaves separately.

PER SERVING Calories 380; Total Carbohydrates 6g; Sugar 2g; Total Fat 16g; Saturated Fat 4g; Sodium 417mg; Protein 50g; Fiber 1g

SALADE NIÇOISE

SERVES 4 ° PREP TIME: 10 MINUTES ° COOK TIME: 15 TO 20 MINUTES

DAIRY-FREE
NUT-FREE
MAKE VEGETARIAN

1 pound small
   waxy potatoes
4 eggs
Sea salt
2 (6- to 8-ounce)
   ahi tuna steaks
3 tablespoons extra-virgin
   olive oil, divided
Freshly ground
   black pepper
1 tablespoon freshly
   squeezed lemon juice
8 cups mixed greens
½ cup niçoise olives

This salad makes an elegant lunch or a nice light dinner. If you cannot find niçoise olives, choose another mild black olive. The fresh tuna should be of the highest quality because it is best served rare or medium-rare, where the center is warmed but still raw.

1. Place the potatoes and eggs in a large pot of water. Season with salt. Bring to a simmer over medium-high heat, cover, set the heat to low, and cook for 10 minutes.

2. With a slotted spoon, transfer the eggs to an ice-water bath to stop the cooking process. When cool, carefully peel and halve each egg. Set aside.

3. Continue cooking the potatoes until they are just tender, about 5 more minutes. Drain the potatoes and transfer them to a cutting board, and cut into 2-inch chunks.

4. Pat the tuna steaks dry with paper towels. Coat the steaks with 1 tablespoon of the olive oil, then season both sides with salt and pepper.

5. Heat a large skillet or sauté pan over medium-high heat until hot, about 2 minutes. Place the tuna steaks in the pan and sear for 1 to 2 minutes on each side. Transfer the tuna to a cutting board and slice on a bias.

6. In a large bowl, whisk the lemon juice and the remaining 2 tablespoons of olive oil. Season with salt and pepper. Add the greens to the bowl and gently toss to coat with the dressing.

7. Evenly divide the greens among 4 serving plates. Top each with potatoes, 2 egg halves, several slices of tuna, and the niçoise olives.

SUBSTITUTION TIP To make this salad vegetarian, omit the tuna and add 2 additional eggs.

PER SERVING Calories 423; Total Carbohydrates 23g; Sugar 3g; Total Fat 22g; Saturated Fat 5g; Sodium 323mg; Protein 34g; Fiber 4g

RICE NOODLE BOWLS

SERVES 4 ° PREP TIME: 10 MINUTES

DAIRY-FREE
EGG-FREE
MAKE NUT-FREE

6 ounces thin rice noodles
Boiling water, for cooking
the rice noodles
¼ cup gluten-free
soy sauce
2 tablespoons freshly
squeezed lime juice
1 tablespoon toasted
sesame oil
1 teaspoon honey,
or brown sugar
1 teaspoon peeled minced
fresh ginger
1 teaspoon minced garlic
⅓ cup canola oil
2 cups sliced
cooked chicken
4 cups mixed lettuces
1 cup fresh herbs, such as
basil, cilantro, and mint
1 cucumber, diced
1 cup roughly chopped
roasted peanuts
(optional)

This tangy vegetable noodle salad is one of my favorite lunchtime treats. It's easy to prepare ahead of time and store the dressing in a glass jar. You can alternate the vegetables based on whatever is fresh in your kitchen.

1. In a heatproof container, cover the rice noodles with boiling water. Rehydrate for 5 minutes or until soft. Drain in a colander, rinse under cool running water, and then drain again thoroughly.

2. In a large sealable jar, whisk the soy sauce, lime juice, sesame oil, honey or brown sugar, ginger, and garlic. Add the canola oil. Seal the lid and shake the jar to emulsify the ingredients.

3. Transfer the noodles to a large bowl. Pour half the dressing over them and gently toss with tongs to coat.

4. Evenly divide the noodles among 4 serving bowls. Top each with chicken, lettuce, herbs, and cucumber.

5. Drizzle with the remaining dressing and top with the roasted peanuts (if using).

SUBSTITUTION TIP For peanut allergies, roughly chopped cashews can be a tasty substitute. For tree nut allergies, use toasted shelled sunflower seeds.

PER SERVING Calories 366; Total Carbohydrates 20g; Sugar 4g; Total Fat 24g; Saturated Fat 2g; Sodium 954mg; Protein 19g; Fiber 3g

EVERYDAY GREEN SALAD

SERVES 1 ∘ PREP TIME: 5 MINUTES

ALLERGEN-FREE
DAIRY-FREE
EGG-FREE
NUT-FREE
ONE POT
MAKE VEGAN

2 tablespoons extra-virgin
olive oil

1 tablespoon red
wine vinegar

Sea salt

Freshly ground
black pepper

2 cups arugula, or
other leafy green

½ cup halved cherry
tomatoes

½ avocado, diced

¾ cup sliced
cooked chicken

I'll be honest; I don't usually consult cookbooks when I cook lunch. I open the refrigerator, reach in for whatever greens I have on hand, add a few seasonal vegetables, and finish with some chicken or whatever protein is left from the night before. Lunch shouldn't be complicated! So, here's my everyday green salad. And yes, I do eat something like this pretty much every day.

1. In a large salad bowl, whisk the olive oil and vinegar until emulsified. Season with salt and pepper.

2. Add the arugula, tomatoes, and avocado. Gently toss to mix.

3. Top with the sliced chicken.

SUBSTITUTION TIP To make this salad vegan, use rinsed, drained chickpeas or another legume in place of the chicken.

PER SERVING Calories 661; Total Carbohydrates 14g; Sugar 4g; Total Fat 52g; Saturated Fat 8g; Sodium 387g; Protein 40g; Fiber 9g

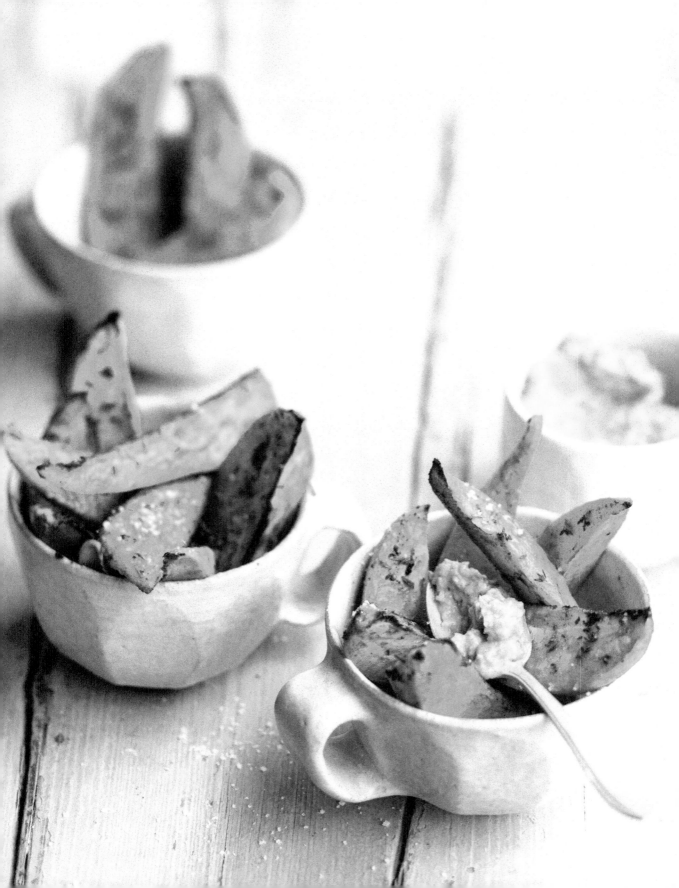

CHAPTER
Four

APPETIZERS
AND SIDES

BAKED SWEET POTATO FRIES

SERVES 4 ° PREP TIME: 5 MINUTES ° COOK TIME: 20 TO 25 MINUTES

ALLERGEN-FREE
NUT-FREE
ONE POT
VEGAN

2 to 3 medium sweet potatoes, unpeeled and scrubbed
1 ½ tablespoons canola oil
¼ teaspoon sea salt

Commercially prepared sweet potato fries often contain gluten because they're coated in wheat flour or cooked in the same fryer with breaded foods. These baked sweet potato fries contain less fat, retain a crisp texture, and are one of my family's favorite appetizers.

1. Preheat the oven to 400°F.

2. Cut the sweet potatoes into thin spears, about ¼ inch thick, and spread them over a rimmed baking sheet.

3. Pour the canola oil over the sweet potatoes and, with your hands, gently toss to coat thoroughly. Spread out the sweet potatoes so all are touching the pan but, as much as possible, not touching each other. Season with the salt.

4. Bake for 20 to 25 minutes, or until the tops of the sweet potatoes are sunken and the bottoms are brown and caramelized.

COOKING TIP To help the fries become crisp and chewy, cut the potatoes into thin slices and don't crowd the pan.

VARIATION TIP If you prefer a "heartier" fry, cut the sweet potatoes into thicker wedges, bake for 35 to 40 minutes, and serve with your favorite dipping sauce.

PER SERVING Calories 223; Total Carbohydrates 42g; Sugar 1g; Total Fat 6g; Saturated Fat 0g; Sodium 131mg; Protein 2g; Fiber 6g

CRISP POTATO SKINS

SERVES 4 ° PREP TIME: 5 MINUTES ° COOK TIME: 25 MINUTES

ALLERGEN-FREE
NUT-FREE
VEGAN

3 medium Russet
  potatoes, scrubbed
¼ cup extra-virgin olive oil
Sea salt
Freshly ground
  black pepper

The microwave isn't usually my first choice for cooking, but it cuts off nearly an hour from the usual time in this recipe. Instead of baking, cook the spuds in the microwave, then crisp the skins in the oven for about 15 minutes.

1. Preheat the oven to 425°F.

2. Prick the potatoes all over with the tines of a fork. Place in a baking dish and microwave for 4 minutes on high. Turn the potatoes over and microwave for 4 minutes more.

3. Use oven-safe mitts to remove the potatoes to a cutting board. Carefully cut each potato lengthwise into 4 wedges. Scoop most of the potato flesh into a bowl and reserve for another use.

4. Place the potato skins on a rimmed baking sheet and brush with the olive oil. Season generously with salt and pepper.

5. Bake for 15 to 17 minutes, until the potato skins are browned and crisp.

INGREDIENT TIP The flavor of the olive oil really shines in this recipe, but if making a nonvegan version, you can also use melted butter.

PER SERVING Calories 163; Total Carbohydrates 13g; Sugar 1g; Total Fat 13g; Saturated Fat 2g; Sodium 63mg; Protein 1g; Fiber 2g

CRUDITÉS PLATTER

SERVES 4 ∘ PREP TIME: 10 MINUTES ∘ COOK TIME: 8 TO 12 MINUTES

ALLERGEN-FREE
NUT-FREE
VEGAN

4 carrots, peeled and
  halved lengthwise
8 ounces green beans
1 bunch broccolini
1 bunch radishes,
  scrubbed and
  greens removed
1 red bell pepper, cored,
  seeded, and thinly sliced

Crudités (cru-dee-tay) sounds way fancier than vegetable platter. But the word really just means rough-cut vegetables. Blanching and shocking vegetables gives them a tender, crisp snap that makes them irresistible, even to children and the usual vegetable skeptics.

1. Fill a large bowl with ice water. Bring a large pot of salted water to a boil over high heat.

2. Add the carrots to the boiling water and cook for 2 to 3 minutes, until bright orange. Using tongs, transfer them to the ice water. When chilled, use a slotted spoon to transfer them to a colander to drain.

3. Add the green beans to the pot of boiling water and cook for 2 to 3 minutes, until bright green and nearly tender. Using tongs, transfer them to the ice water, adding more ice if needed. When chilled, use a slotted spoon to transfer them to the colander to drain.

4. Add the broccolini to the pot of boiling water and cook for 2 to 3 minutes until bright green and nearly tender. Using tongs, transfer them to the ice water, adding more ice if needed. When chilled, use a slotted spoon to transfer them to the colander to drain.

5. Arrange the blanched vegetables on a serving platter along with the radishes and red pepper strips.

COOKING TIP Prepare this recipe ahead of time so it's ready to snack on when you're preparing the main meal.

PER SERVING Calories 63; Total Carbohydrates 14g; Sugar 6g; Total Fat 0g; Saturated Fat 0g; Sodium 58mg; Protein 3g; Fiber 5g

ROASTED VEGETABLES
with Basil Oil

SERVES 4 ° PREP TIME: 5 MINUTES ° COOK TIME: 20 TO 25 MINUTES

ALLERGEN-FREE
NUT-FREE
VEGAN

4 carrots, halved
  lengthwise and cut
  into 2-inch pieces
1 small red onion, cut
  into wedges
1 zucchini, halved
  lengthwise and cut
  into 2-inch pieces
2 yellow potatoes,
  quartered
6 tablespoons extra-virgin
  olive oil, divided
Sea salt
Freshly ground
  black pepper
1 cup fresh basil leaves
Zest of 1 lemon
Juice of 1 lemon
1 garlic clove

This was one of the first dishes I made when my family and I moved to Santa Barbara. I picked the most colorful vegetables I could find at the farmers' market and prepared this simple sauce to drizzle over the top.

1. Preheat the oven to 425°F.

2. On a rimmed baking sheet, spread out the carrots, onion, zucchini, and potatoes. Drizzle with 1½ tablespoons of the olive oil. Using your hands, gently toss to coat. Season with salt and pepper.

3. Roast, uncovered, for 20 to 25 minutes, until the vegetables are tender and begin to caramelize.

4. Meanwhile, in a blender, combine the remaining 4½ tablespoons olive oil, the basil, lemon zest, lemon juice, and garlic. Purée until smooth. Alternatively, combine the ingredients in a medium bowl and purée with an immersion blender. Season with salt.

5. Transfer the roasted vegetables to a serving platter and pour the basil oil over them. Serve hot or warm.

SUBSTITUTION TIP Use roughly chopped carrot tops in place of the basil if you purchase whole carrots with tops.

PER SERVING Calories 296; Total Carbohydrates 26g; Sugar 6g; Total Fat 21g; Saturated Fat 3g; Sodium 113; Protein 3g; Fiber 5g

ROASTED CHICKPEAS

SERVES 6 ° PREP TIME: 5 MINUTES ° COOK TIME: 20 TO 25 MINUTES

ALLERGEN-FREE
NUT-FREE
ONE POT
VEGAN

2 (15-ounce) cans
  chickpeas, rinsed and
  thoroughly drained
3 tablespoons extra-virgin
  olive oil
Sea salt
Freshly ground
  black pepper
1 teaspoon smoked
  paprika
½ teaspoon ground cumin
1 garlic clove, minced

Potato chips have met their match in this healthy, fiber-rich appetizer. Toss the chickpeas with the spices and garlic after roasting to prevent the garlic from burning.

1. Preheat the oven to 425°F.

2. Pat the chickpeas dry with a clean kitchen towel or paper towels, and spread them out over a rimmed baking sheet.

3. Drizzle with the olive oil and gently toss to coat. Season with salt and pepper.

4. Roast, uncovered, for 20 to 25 minutes, or until the chickpeas are crisp. Shake the pan gently once or twice during the baking time so the chickpeas roast evenly. Transfer to a large bowl.

5. Sprinkle the roasted chickpeas with the paprika, cumin, and garlic. Toss to coat and serve hot.

COOKING TIP Play around with the flavors. Chickpeas are also delicious with fresh rosemary, thyme, and lemon zest.

PER SERVING Calories 320; Total Carbohydrates 43g; Sugar 8g; Total Fat 11g; Saturated Fat 1g; Sodium 57mg; Protein 14g; Fiber 13g

SPINACH AND ARTICHOKE DIP

SERVES 6 ° PREP TIME: 5 MINUTES ° COOK TIME: 8 TO 11 MINUTES

EGG-FREE
NUT-FREE
ONE POT
VEGETARIAN

4 cups fresh spinach,
  roughly chopped
3 garlic cloves, minced
1 teaspoon extra-virgin
  olive oil
8 ounces full-fat
  cream cheese
½ cup full-fat sour cream
½ cup shredded
  Parmesan cheese
½ cup shredded
  mozzarella cheese
1 (15-ounce) can
  artichoke hearts,
  roughly chopped
Sea salt
Freshly ground
  black pepper

Spinach and artichoke dip is ubiquitous on appetizer menus, but it typically contains wheat as a thickener and stabilizer. This version is just as flavorful but deliciously gluten-free. Serve with root vegetable chips for a burst of color and added nutrients.

1. In a large skillet or sauté pan over medium-low heat, cook the spinach and garlic with the olive oil for 5 minutes, tossing regularly, until the spinach releases most of its liquid. Transfer to a colander to cool and drain.

2. Pour out any liquid remaining in the skillet and return it to the heat.

3. Add the cream cheese and sour cream to the skillet, and cook for 1 to 2 minutes until softened.

4. Stir in the Parmesan cheese and mozzarella cheese, and cook for 1 to 2 minutes, until just melted.

5. Fold in the artichoke hearts and cooked spinach and garlic. Cook for 1 to 2 minutes until just heated through. Season with salt and pepper.

COOKING TIP Low-fat dairy products are a tempting substitution for whole milk and full-fat cheese, but fat helps dairy remain stable during cooking, so experiment carefully.

PER SERVING Calories 277; Total Carbohydrates 11g; Sugar 1g; Total Fat 22g; Saturated Fat 13g; Sodium 388mg; Protein 12g; Fiber 4g

SMOKY BACON
and Roasted Corn Dip

SERVES 6 ° PREP TIME: 5 MINUTES ° COOK TIME: 15 TO 18 MINUTES

EGG-FREE
NUT-FREE
ONE POT
MAKE VEGETARIAN

2 applewood smoked
  bacon slices, roughly
  chopped
1 teaspoon minced garlic
1 scallion, white and green
  parts, thinly sliced
1 cup frozen roasted
  corn kernels, thawed
1 plum tomato,
  seeded and diced
1 teaspoon smoked
  paprika
8 ounces full-fat
  cream cheese
½ cup full-fat sour cream
½ cup shredded pepper
  Jack cheese
½ cup shredded
  mozzarella cheese
Sea salt
Freshly ground
  black pepper

This smoky, cheesy dip is perfect for dipping the
Crudités Platter (page 82) or corn chips. It's also
delicious spooned over the Crisp Potato Skins
(page 81) for a complete meal.

1. In a large skillet or sauté pan over medium-low heat,
   cook the bacon for 10 minutes, until it renders most of its
   fat. Use a slotted spoon to transfer it to a paper towel to
   drain. Leave the fat in the skillet.

2. Add the garlic and scallion to the bacon fat. Cook for
   about 1 minute until fragrant.

3. Stir in the corn, tomato, and paprika. Cook for about
   1 minute, until just heated through.

4. Add the cream cheese and sour cream to the skillet.
   Cook for 1 to 2 minutes until softened.

5. Stir in the pepper Jack cheese and mozzarella cheese,
   and cook for 1 to 2 minutes more until melted.

6. Fold in the cooked bacon. Cook for 1 to 2 minutes more,
   until just heated through. Season with salt and pepper.

SUBSTITUTION TIP For a vegetarian version, omit the bacon
and cook the garlic and scallion in 1 tablespoon of melted butter.
Optional: add ¼ teaspoon of liquid smoke.

PER SERVING Calories 339; Total Carbohydrates 8g; Sugar 1g;
Total Fat 28g; Saturated Fat 16g; Sodium 605; Protein 15g; Fiber 1g

PROSCIUTTO-WRAPPED DATES

SERVES 6 ∘ PREP TIME: 5 MINUTES ∘ COOK TIME: 15 TO 18 MINUTES

EGG-FREE
ONE POT

12 Medjool dates, pitted
12 blanched slivered
almonds
2 ounces hard cheese,
such as Manchego
or Parmesan, cut
into 12 pieces
6 slices prosciutto,
halved lengthwise

This appetizer manages to be both simple and sophisticated at once. Preparation involves more assembly than real cooking, but the results are impressive and addicting! If you can find Marcona almonds, which are softer and sweeter, use those in place of the slivered almonds and serve the remaining almonds as a side dish.

1. Preheat the oven to 350°F.

2. Line a rimmed baking sheet with parchment paper.

3. Stuff each date with 1 almond and 1 piece of cheese and fold together to enclose.

4. Wrap each stuffed date with a prosciutto strip and place it seam-side down on the prepared sheet.

5. Bake for 15 to 18 minutes, until the prosciutto is gently browned. Let rest for 5 minutes before serving.

SERVING TIP Remind your guests that the dates are pitted but they do contain a crunchy almond, which may be mistaken for a pit.

PER SERVING Calories 153; Total Carbohydrates 14g; Sugar 11g; Total Fat 6g; Saturated Fat 2g; Sodium 599mg; Protein 13g; Fiber 2g

GRAIN-FREE BREADSTICKS

MAKES 6 (6-INCH) BREADSTICKS ° PREP TIME: 5 MINUTES
COOK TIME: 12 TO 14 MINUTES

DAIRY-FREE
VEGETARIAN

¾ cup finely ground
  blanched almond flour
½ cup tapioca
  flour (starch)
¼ teaspoon sea salt
1 teaspoon aluminum-
  free, double-acting
  baking powder
1 egg
1 tablespoon extra-virgin
  olive oil

Most breadstick recipes rely on yeast and at least
45 minutes of rising time, but these are leavened
with baking powder and rise in just 14 minutes in
the oven.

1. Preheat the oven to 350°F.

2. Line a baking sheet with parchment paper.

3. In a medium bowl, mix the almond flour, tapioca flour,
   salt, and baking powder.

4. Whisk in the egg and olive oil until combined.

5. Form the mixture into 6 small balls. Roll each ball into
   a long spear with the heel of your hand, and carefully
   transfer to the prepared pan.

6. Bake for 12 to 14 minutes, until just beginning to brown.

COOKING TIP To make garlic breadsticks, brush the tops with
1 tablespoon of melted butter and sprinkle with ½ teaspoon of
garlic salt.

PER SERVING Calories 145; Total Carbohydrates 14g; Sugar 1g; Total Fat 9g;
Saturated Fat 1g; Sodium 89mg; Protein 3g; Fiber 2g

STUFFED MUSHROOMS

SERVES 4 ° PREP TIME: 5 MINUTES ° COOK TIME: 20 MINUTES

NUT-FREE
VEGETARIAN

8 ounces cream cheese,
  at room temperature
½ cup shredded
  Parmesan cheese
½ cup gluten-free
  bread crumbs
1 garlic clove, minced
1 teaspoon minced
  fresh rosemary
1 teaspoon fresh
  thyme leaves
¼ teaspoon freshly
  ground black pepper
8 ounces button or cremini
  mushrooms, stemmed

Sometimes I like to serve nothing but appetizers for dinner. We call it "tapas," but really it's just a collection of my favorite side dishes. These stuffed mushrooms are flavorful and super easy to whip up when you're making several things. Alternatively, use meaty portobello mushrooms and make the dish into an entrée served with a side salad and some sautéed green beans.

1. Preheat the oven to 425°F.

2. In a small bowl, mix the cream cheese, Parmesan cheese, bread crumbs, garlic, rosemary, thyme, and pepper.

3. Fill the mushrooms, evenly dividing the mixture among them and place them, filling-side up, on a baking sheet.

4. Bake for 20 minutes, or until the tops are golden brown and bubbling.

INGREDIENT TIP You can purchase gluten-free bread crumbs or make your own. Toast 1 slice of gluten-free bread and then pulse it a few times in a spice grinder or food processor until coarsely ground.

PER SERVING Calories 312; Total Carbohydrates 14g; Sugar 2g; Total Fat 24g; Saturated Fat 15g; Sodium 402mg; Protein 13g; Fiber 5g

BAKED CHICKEN
and Cheese Taquitos

SERVES 6 ° PREP TIME: 10 MINUTES ° COOK TIME: 15 TO 17 MINUTES

EGG-FREE
NUT-FREE

8 ounces cream cheese,
  at room temperature
1 cup shredded sharp
  Cheddar cheese
1 cup shredded cooked
  skinless chicken breast
1 tablespoon minced
  jalapeño pepper
1 teaspoon ground cumin
1 teaspoon minced garlic
2 tablespoons
  minced onion
12 gluten-free
  corn tortillas

Whether you're looking for a healthy snack for game day or an easy dinner for the kids, these chicken and cheese taquitos are perfect. Because they're not cooked in a deep fryer, they're healthier than taquitos you might get at a restaurant. Even more important, you can ensure they're completely gluten-free.

1. Preheat the oven to 425°F.

2. Line a rimmed baking sheet with parchment paper.

3. In a medium bowl, stir together the cream cheese, Cheddar cheese, chicken, jalapeño, cumin, garlic, and onion.

4. Warm each tortilla for 10 seconds in the microwave. Fill with ¼ cup of the cheese mixture. Roll the tortilla, leaving the ends open, and place them seam-side down on the prepared sheet.

5. Bake for 15 to 17 minutes until gently browned and crisp.

INGREDIENT TIP Always read the label when purchasing corn tortillas to make sure they are gluten-free. Many artisan varieties use wheat flour to produce a pliable texture.

PER SERVING Calories 208; Total Carbohydrates 10g; Sugar 1g; Total Fat 16g; Saturated Fat 10g; Sodium 268mg; Protein 8g; Fiber 1g

HERBED GOAT CHEESE
and Sun-Dried Tomato Bites

SERVES 6 ° PREP TIME: 10 MINUTES

EGG-FREE
NUT-FREE
VEGETARIAN

6 ounces fresh
  goat cheese
2 tablespoons minced
  fresh herbs, such as
  parsley, basil, tarragon,
  and thyme
8 ounces gluten-free
  crackers
½ cup oil-packed
  sliced sun-dried
  tomatoes, drained

The flavor combination of these simple appetizers is mind blowing. So is their simplicity. When purchasing crackers to go with this recipe, opt for plain salted ones and crackers flavored with olive oil or herbs. This recipe also works exceptionally well with gluten-free crostini.

1. In a small bowl, stir together the goat cheese and fresh herbs.

2. Spread the herbed cheese on the crackers and then top each with a slice of sun-dried tomato.

SUBSTITUTION TIP If you're not a fan of the pungent flavor of goat cheese, use cream cheese.

PER SERVING Calories 323; Total Carbohydrates 25g; Sugar 2g; Total Fat 20g; Saturated Fat 8g; Sodium 419mg; Protein 12g; Fiber 1g

TOMATO, SHALLOT,
and Mint Salad

SERVES 4 ° PREP TIME: 5 MINUTES ° REST TIME: 20 MINUTES

**2 pounds ripe tomatoes,
heirloom if available,
cored, and cut
horizontally into
¼-inch-thick slices**

**5 fresh mint leaves,
thinly sliced**

2 shallots, thinly sliced

**2 tablespoons extra-virgin
olive oil**

**1 teaspoon red
wine vinegar**

Sea salt

**Freshly ground
black pepper**

Don't you love recipes that benefit from being forgotten about? It's so nice to prepare something, and then have it improve while you get on with other kitchen tasks. The salt in this salad draws out the liquid from the tomatoes, enriching their flavor and integrating it with the shallots and mint.

1. Spread the tomato slices on a serving platter. Top with the mint leaves and shallots. Drizzle with the olive oil and vinegar. Season with salt and pepper.

2. Let rest at room temperature for 20 minutes before serving.

INGREDIENT TIP Prepare this recipe in the summer when tomatoes are at their peak freshness and can be found easily at the farmers' market.

PER SERVING Calories 105; Total Carbohydrates 10g; Sugar 6g; Total Fat 8g; Saturated Fat 1g; Sodium 70mg; Protein 2g; Fiber 3g

CUCUMBER, AVOCADO, and Watermelon Salad

SERVES 4 ∘ PREP TIME: 1O MINUTES

4 cups cubed watermelon

2 large tomatoes, cored and diced

1 English cucumber, cut into ½-inch cubes

2 fresh basil leaves, minced

2 fresh mint leaves, minced

1 tablespoon red wine vinegar

1 tablespoon extra-virgin olive oil

Sea salt

Freshly ground black pepper

1 avocado, diced

In the summertime, these ingredients are on my counter and in my fruit basket at all times, so this salad comes together with only a modicum of effort. Okay, I guess it does require some self-restraint to not eat half of it while I'm making it.

1. In a large serving bowl, combine the watermelon, tomatoes, cucumber, basil, and mint.

2. Drizzle with the vinegar and olive oil. Season with salt and pepper.

3. Add the avocado and stir very gently to combine.

SERVING TIP If you're preparing this salad ahead of time, add the avocado just before serving.

PER SERVING Calories 201; Total Carbohydrates 21g; Sugar 13g; Total Fat 14g; Saturated Fat 3g; Sodium 68mg; Protein 3g; Fiber 5g

QUINOA, CHERRY, and Almond Salad

SERVES 4 ∘ PREP TIME: 5 MINUTES ∘ COOK TIME: 20 MINUTES

ONE POT
VEGAN

1 cup quinoa, rinsed
  and drained
2 cups water
Sea salt
2 tablespoons extra-virgin
  olive oil
1 tablespoon balsamic
  vinegar
2 cups roughly chopped
  fresh baby spinach
½ cup dried cherries,
  roughly chopped
½ cup slivered almonds
Freshly ground
  black pepper

Quinoa, almonds, and spinach make for a filling side dish that is rich in protein and complex carbohydrates. It makes a delicious lunch entrée, as well.

1. In a medium pot over medium heat, combine the quinoa, water, and a pinch salt. Bring to a simmer, reduce the heat to low, cover, and cook for about 20 minutes, until the quinoa is cooked through. Remove from the heat and fluff with a fork.

2. Gently stir in the olive oil and vinegar to combine.

3. While the quinoa is hot, stir in the spinach, cherries, and almonds. Let the spinach wilt.

4. Season with salt and pepper. Serve warm or cover and chill.

INGREDIENT TIP Look for unsweetened dried cherries. Or, make your own by pitting and halving fresh cherries and then drying them in a dehydrator for 12 hours.

PER SERVING Calories 297; Total Carbohydrates 32g; Sugar 1g; Total Fat 16g; Saturated Fat 2g; Sodium 73mg; Protein 9g; Fiber 5g

AVOCADO, BLACK BEAN,
and Quinoa Salad

SERVES 4 ° PREP TIME: 10 MINUTES ° COOK TIME: 20 MINUTES

ALLERGEN-FREE
NUT-FREE
ONE POT
VEGAN

1 cup quinoa, rinsed
and drained

2 cups vegetable broth,
or water

1 (15-ounce) can
black beans, rinsed
and drained

1 pint grape
tomatoes, halved

2 avocados, pitted
and diced

½ cup roughly chopped
fresh cilantro

2 garlic cloves, minced

2 tablespoons freshly
squeezed lime juice

2 tablespoons extra-virgin
olive oil

½ teaspoon ground cumin

¼ teaspoon sea salt

⅛ teaspoon
cayenne pepper

I love the tangy lime and cilantro dressing that coats this hearty quinoa salad. Like the Quinoa, Cherry, and Almond Salad (page 94), this makes a delicious side dish or lunch entrée.

1. In a medium pot over medium-high heat, combine the quinoa and vegetable broth. Bring to a simmer, reduce the heat to low, cover, and cook for about 20 minutes, or until the quinoa is cooked through. Fluff with a fork.

2. Stir in the black beans, tomatoes, and avocado.

3. In a small bowl, whisk the cilantro, garlic, lime juice, olive oil, cumin, salt, and cayenne pepper. Pour the dressing over the quinoa and gently stir to combine.

4. Serve warm or cover and chill.

INGREDIENT TIP If you're serving this to children, omit or reduce the cayenne pepper.

PER SERVING Calories 635; Total Carbohydrates 76g; Sugar 4g; Total Fat 30g; Saturated Fat 6g; Sodium 134mg; Protein 21g; Fiber 20g

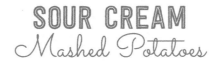

SOUR CREAM
Mashed Potatoes

SERVES 4 ° PREP TIME: 5 MINUTES ° COOK TIME: 15 MINUTES

EGG-FREE
NUT-FREE
ONE POT
VEGETARIAN

2½ pounds Yukon Gold
   potatoes, quartered
8 ounces full-fat
   sour cream
2 tablespoons butter
½ to 1 cup milk
2 tablespoons minced
   fresh chives (optional)

Mashed potatoes go with everything and, as such, often get less of our attention, ending up bland and pasty. This version uses sour cream for a little tang. If you don't have a potato ricer, you can use an immersion blender or a classic potato masher.

1. Place the potatoes in a large pot of salted water. Bring to a boil over high heat and cook for about 15 minutes, until the potatoes are fork-tender. Drain the potatoes thoroughly, then pass them through a potato ricer into the same pot.

2. Stir in the sour cream and butter. Add enough milk to thin the potatoes to your desired consistency.

3. Serve garnished with fresh chives (if using).

COOKING TIP If you use a potato ricer, you do not need to peel the potatoes.

PER SERVING Calories 413; Total Carbohydrates 55g; Sugar 5g; Total Fat 19g; Saturated Fat 11g; Sodium 128mg; Protein 10g; Fiber 4g

ROASTED CAULIFLOWER

SERVES 2 TO 4 ° PREP TIME: 5 MINUTES ° COOK TIME: 25 MINUTES

ALLERGEN-FREE
NUT-FREE
VEGAN

1 head cauliflower, cored
  and broken into florets
¼ cup extra-virgin olive oil
1 tablespoon
  minced garlic
Zest of 1 lemon
¼ cup minced
  fresh parsley
Sea salt
Freshly ground
  black pepper
Juice of 1 lemon

The first time Cole saw this appetizer, he laughed and said, "That looks like a polar bear butt!" So that's what he calls it now. And, hey, if it gets him to eat another vegetable, I'm all for funny-sounding nicknames!

1. Preheat the oven to 425°F.

2. In a large mixing bowl, combine the cauliflower, olive oil, garlic, lemon zest, and parsley. With your hands, mix to coat all the cauliflower pieces. Spread the mixture onto a rimmed baking sheet. Season generously with salt and pepper.

3. Roast, uncovered, for 25 minutes, or until the cauliflower is deeply browned on the bottom and wilted.

4. Sprinkle with the lemon juice and serve.

COOKING TIP You can prepare this all on the baking sheet, instead of mixing the cauliflower in the bowl. However, be aware that some garlic pieces might stick to the pan and burn, so avoid serving any burnt bits.

PER SERVING Calories 258; Total Carbohydrates 9g; Sugar 3g; Total Fat 25g; Saturated Fat 4g; Sodium 162mg; Protein 3g; Fiber 4g

CREAMY POLENTA

SERVES 4 ∘ PREP TIME: 5 MINUTES ∘ COOK TIME: 15 MINUTES

EGG-FREE

NUT-FREE

ONE POT

VEGETARIAN

MAKE DAIRY-FREE

MAKE VEGAN

3 cups water, or low-
sodium chicken broth
Sea salt
1 cup yellow cornmeal
2 tablespoons butter
¼ cup shredded
Parmesan cheese

You can buy prepared polenta in plastic packages from the grocery store. It is sliceable and can be panfried. Homemade polenta is entirely different. It has a creamy consistency, somewhere between mashed potatoes and Cream of Wheat. It takes a little more attention than rice, but cooks quickly and is worth the extra effort.

1. In a medium pot over medium-low heat, bring the water to a simmer with a generous pinch salt added.

2. Whisking constantly, pour in the cornmeal in a slow, thin, steady stream.

3. Reduce the heat to low and continue stirring for about 15 minutes until the mixture is thick.

4. Stir in the butter and Parmesan cheese.

SUBSTITUTION TIP For a dairy-free and vegan polenta, use a vegan butter substitute and skip the Parmesan cheese.

PER SERVING Calories 184; Total Carbohydrates 24g; Sugar 0g; Total Fat 8g; Saturated Fat 5g; Sodium 176mg; Protein 5g; Fiber 2g

SPAGHETTI SQUASH
Noodles

SERVES 4 ° PREP TIME: 5 MINUTES ° COOK TIME: 25 MINUTES

ALLERGEN-FREE
NUT-FREE
ONE POT
VEGAN

1 medium spaghetti
squash, cut into 1-inch-
thick rings, seeds and
membranes scooped out
1 tablespoon extra-virgin
olive oil

The first time I tried spaghetti squash, my expecta-tions were pretty low. How could a humble squash produce long, thin strands of pasta? Needless to say, I was pleasantly surprised at how closely the vegetable resembled traditional spaghetti noodles. Here's the trick, though—slice the squash crosswise into rings, not lengthwise. This will produce the longest strands.

1. Preheat the oven to 350°F.

2. Line a rimmed baking sheet with parchment paper.

3. Spread the spaghetti squash rings on the prepared sheet, brush with the olive oil, and bake for 25 minutes, or until soft.

4. With a fork, gently peel away the long shreds of squash.

SERVING TIP Serve the cooked spaghetti squash with Meat Lover's Meatballs (page 148) or Cheese Sauce (White Sauce, Variation Tip with cheese, page 214) and leftover Basic Roast Chicken (page 128).

PER SERVING Calories 69; Total Carbohydrates 9g; Sugar 0g; Total Fat 4g; Saturated Fat 1g; Sodium 21mg; Protein 1g; Fiber 0g

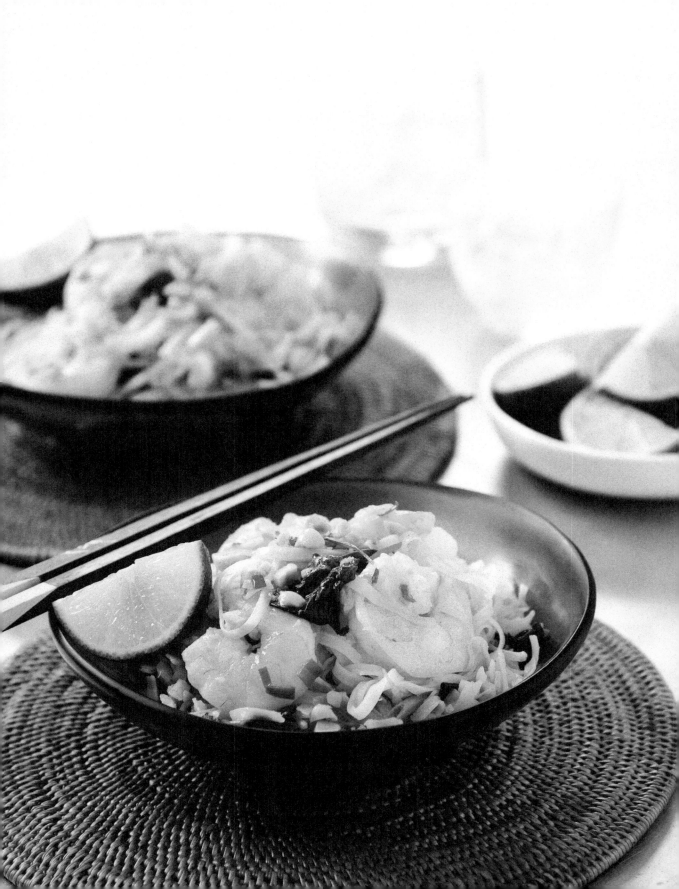

CHAPTER
Five

FISH AND SEAFOOD

PAN-SEARED SALMON
with Orange-Fennel Slaw

SERVES 4 ° PREP TIME: 10 MINUTES ° COOK TIME: 6 TO 8 MINUTES

4 (6- to 8-ounce)
  salmon fillets
3 tablespoons extra-virgin
  olive oil, divided
Sea salt
Freshly ground
  black pepper
1 orange
1 teaspoon red
  wine vinegar
1 teaspoon honey
1 tablespoon
  minced shallot
1 fennel bulb, cored
  and very thinly sliced
2 cups mixed baby greens

The flavors of this salad are bright and addicting, and really take center stage in this recipe. The cooking time for the fish is minimal—it is really about preparation. If you can find microgreens, they provide a beautiful contrast of flavor and texture in the salad.

1. Pat the salmon fillets dry with a paper towel, and coat them with 1 tablespoon of the olive oil. Season generously on both sides with salt and pepper.

2. Heat a large skillet or sauté pan over medium-high heat. Sear the salmon fillets for 3 to 4 minutes on each side, or until the fish flakes easily with a fork but is still a deeper shade of pink on the inside. It will continue to cook after it is out of the pan.

3. While the salmon is cooking, zest the orange with a zester or a paring knife into a salad bowl, cutting only strips of the orange part of the outer peel, not the white pith. Remove the rest of the white pith and discard. Working over the bowl, slice down along the side of each orange membrane, freeing the orange segments and allowing the juices to drip into the bowl. Set the orange segments aside. Squeeze the remaining juice from the membranes into the bowl.

4. Add the remaining 2 tablespoons olive oil, the vinegar, honey, and shallot to the bowl. Season with salt and pepper and whisk to emulsify the mixture.

5. Add the fennel and greens to the salad bowl and gently toss to coat with the dressing.

6. Evenly divide the salad among 4 serving plates. Garnish with the orange segments, and top each salad with a seared salmon fillet.

COOKING TIP Use a vegetable peeler to cut the fennel into long, thin shavings.

PER SERVING Calories 380; Total Carbohydrates 15g; Sugar 6g; Total Fat 21g; Saturated Fat 3g; Sodium 184mg; Protein 36g; Fiber 4g

PESTO SALMON
with Asparagus

SERVES 4 ∘ PREP TIME: 5 MINUTES ∘ COOK TIME: 15 MINUTES

1 bunch asparagus,
  woody ends trimmed
1 tablespoon extra-virgin
  olive oil
Sea salt
Freshly ground
  black pepper
1 ½ pounds salmon,
  ideally one thick fillet
¼ cup prepared pesto

I wrote a book devoted to meals that could be made solely on a baking sheet. The trick was combining ingredients that had similar cooking times. However, cooking time for salmon varies widely based on the thickness of the fillet. An evenly cut continuous fillet makes it easier to ensure the entire piece of fish is uniformly cooked.

1. Preheat the oven to 375°F.

2. Line a baking sheet with parchment paper.

3. Coat the asparagus with the olive oil and season generously with salt and pepper. Spread the asparagus spears out on the baking sheet, leaving space in the center of the pan for the salmon.

4. Coat the salmon with the pesto and place it on the pan in the center.

5. Roast, uncovered, for 15 minutes, until the salmon is not quite cooked through; it should still be deep pink in the center, but flake with a fork. It will continue cooking after it emerges from the oven.

SUBSTITUTION TIP To make this recipe dairy-free, make your own pesto by combining 2 tablespoons toasted pine nuts, 1 cup fresh basil, 1 garlic clove, 1 teaspoon freshly squeezed lemon juice, and 2 tablespoons extra-virgin olive oil. Purée in a blender until mostly smooth and season with salt. Makes about ½ cup.

PER SERVING Calories 335; Total Carbohydrates 4g; Sugar 2g; Total Fat 21g; Saturated Fat 3g; Sodium 230mg; Protein 36g; Fiber 2g

HAZELNUT-CRUSTED HALIBUT
with Honeyed Peaches

SERVES 4 ∘ PREP TIME: 10 MINUTES ∘ COOK TIME: 15 MINUTES

DAIRY-FREE
EGG-FREE
SPLURGE-WORTHY

4 peaches, peeled
  and sliced
2 tablespoons honey
1 teaspoon red
  wine vinegar
1 teaspoon minced
  fresh rosemary
½ cup ground hazelnuts
½ teaspoon sea salt
¼ teaspoon freshly
  ground black pepper
4 (5- to 6-ounce)
  halibut fillets
2 tablespoons extra-virgin
  olive oil, divided

Hazelnut flour is a gluten-free baking flour with a texture similar to almond flour. I make my own by grinding toasted hazelnuts in a clean coffee grinder.

1. In a small saucepan over medium-low heat, combine the peaches, honey, vinegar, and rosemary. Bring to a gentle simmer then reduce the heat to low. Cook for about 10 minutes, stirring frequently, until thick and slightly broken down.

2. While the peaches simmer, preheat a cast iron or stainless-steel skillet over medium-high heat, for 2 to 3 minutes.

3. In a shallow dish, mix the hazelnuts, salt, and pepper.

4. Pat the fillets dry with paper towels. Coat them with 1 tablespoon of olive oil and then press both sides into the hazelnut mixture.

5. Add the remaining tablespoon olive oil to the hot skillet and tilt the pan to coat the bottom.

6. Place the fillets in the hot skillet and cook for 4 minutes on each side until a brown crust forms and the fish flakes easily with a fork.

7. Serve with the honeyed peaches on the side.

SUBSTITUTION TIP Halibut is an expensive, mild-flavored white fish. For a less expensive fish, choose cod. It has a more distinct flavor and less meaty flesh, but will work well in this recipe.

PER SERVING Calories 381; Total Carbohydrates 20g; Sugar 17g; Total Fat 15g; Saturated Fat 2g; Sodium 383mg; Protein 44g; Fiber 3g

FISH AND CHIPS

SERVES 4 ° PREP TIME: 10 MINUTES ° COOK TIME: 25 MINUTES

DAIRY-FREE
NUT-FREE

2 large Russet potatoes, scrubbed, and cut into ¼-inch-wide spears
2 tablespoons extra-virgin olive oil
½ teaspoon sea salt, divided
1 ½ cups gluten-free bread crumbs
¼ teaspoon garlic powder
Pinch cayenne pepper
2 eggs
1 ½ pounds cod fillets, cut into 1-inch-thick spears

If you're looking for deep-fried fish dripping with oil and served in a newspaper-lined basket, hit up a local seafood joint. These baked fish and chips are a far healthier option, with a much lower risk of burning down your kitchen. Trust me.

1. Preheat the oven to 425°F.

2. Line a rimmed baking sheet with parchment paper.

3. Spread the potato spears on the pan and drizzle with the olive oil. Gently toss to coat. Season with ¼ teaspoon of the salt. Bake for 15 minutes.

4. Meanwhile, in a shallow dish, mix the bread crumbs, the remaining ¼ teaspoon salt, garlic powder, and cayenne pepper.

5. Thoroughly whisk the eggs in a separate shallow dish.

6. Dip the cod fillets into the seasoned bread crumbs mixture, then dip them into the egg, and then dip, once more, into the bread crumbs.

7. Remove the potatoes from the oven and add the coated fish to the pan. Bake for 10 minutes more, or until the fish is cooked through and the potatoes are browned.

SERVING TIP For a classic side dish, whip up a simple coleslaw with ¼ cup mayonnaise, 1 tablespoon freshly squeezed lemon juice, and 4 cups shredded cabbage. To keep it crisp, dress the salad just before serving.

PER SERVING Calories 504; Total Carbohydrates 46g; Sugar 4g; Total Fat 13g; Saturated Fat 3g; Sodium 700mg; Protein 49g; Fiber 4g

FISH VERA CRUZ

SERVES 4 ∘ PREP TIME: 5 MINUTES ∘ COOK TIME: 20 MINUTES

DAIRY-FREE
EGG-FREE
NUT-FREE
ONE POT

2 tablespoons extra-virgin
   olive oil
1 red onion, halved
   and thinly sliced
2 garlic cloves, minced
⅛ teaspoon red
   pepper flakes
2 tablespoons capers,
   rinsed and drained
¼ cup pitted green olives
1 (15-ounce) can plum
   tomatoes, drained
   and hand crushed
1 tablespoon red
   wine vinegar
1 teaspoon minced
   fresh rosemary
1½ pounds flaky white
   fish, such as red snapper
   or sea bass
Sea salt
Freshly ground
   black pepper
¼ cup minced fresh parsley
1 lemon, cut into 4 wedges

This is one of my favorite fish preparation methods because I love the balance of spicy red pepper flakes, briny capers and olives, and sweet plum tomatoes. Use whatever flaky white fish looks best at the market. The recipe is naturally gluten-free and goes well with oven-roasted potatoes.

1. In a large skillet or sauté pan over medium heat, heat the olive oil. Add the onion, garlic, and red pepper flakes. Cook for about 5 minutes, stirring frequently, until the onion is somewhat softened.

2. Stir in the capers, olives, tomatoes, vinegar, and rosemary. Simmer for 5 minutes, uncovered.

3. Add the fish to the pan and season with salt and pepper. Simmer for 5 minutes, then flip the fish and continue cooking for about 4 minutes more, until the fish is cooked through.

4. Plate each fish fillet and top with a generous spoonful of the tomato mixture.

5. Shower with fresh parsley and garnish with a lemon wedge.

INGREDIENT TIP If tomatoes are in season, use fresh vine-ripened tomatoes. Cut into quarters and use as instructed.

PER SERVING Calories 315; Total Carbohydrates 10g; Sugar 4g; Total Fat 11g; Saturated Fat 2g; Sodium 657mg; Protein 43g; Fiber 3g

BAJA FISH TACOS

SERVES 4 ∘ PREP TIME: 15 MINUTES ∘ COOK TIME: 8 MINUTES

NUT-FREE

2 tablespoons extra-virgin
   olive oil
Zest of 1 lime
Juice of 1 lime
1 teaspoon ground cumin
1 teaspoon ancho
   chile powder
¼ teaspoon sea salt
⅛ teaspoon
   cayenne pepper
1 pound mahi mahi, cut
   into 4-inch-long pieces
½ cup mayonnaise
½ cup sour cream
¼ cup minced
   fresh cilantro
16 gluten-free
   corn tortillas
1 cup shredded cabbage
½ red onion, thinly sliced
1 cup store-bought gluten-
   free roasted tomato salsa

If you have tried to make fish tacos at home but find yourself disappointed with the results, I feel your pain! I spent years trying to re-create the fish tacos I enjoyed at trendy beachside restaurants and have come to discover that it's all in the sauce. If you prefer breaded fish tacos, follow the instructions in the recipe for Fish and Chips (page 106).

1. In a large, nonreactive dish, whisk the olive oil, lime zest, lime juice, cumin, ancho chile powder, salt, and cayenne pepper. Add the mahi mahi to this mixture, turn to coat, and refrigerate for 10 minutes.

2. In a small jar, whisk the mayonnaise, sour cream, and cilantro. Cover and refrigerate until ready to serve.

3. Heat a large skillet or sauté pan over medium-high heat until hot. Remove the mahi mahi from the marinade, add to the skillet, and panfry for 3 to 4 minutes on each side, or until it flakes easily with a fork.

4. Evenly divide the fish among the tortillas. Top each taco with some of the shredded cabbage, onion, and salsa. Finish with a dollop of the cilantro sauce.

INGREDIENT TIP The Monterey Bay Aquarium recommends US pole-caught mahi mahi as a "best choice" for protecting the ocean's health. For more recommendations, visit SeafoodWatch.org.

PER SERVING Calories 602; Total Carbohydrates 58g; Sugar 6g; Total Fat 27g; Saturated Fat 7g; Sodium 878mg; Protein 36g; Fiber 8g

CLASSIC CRAB CAKES

SERVES 2 TO 4 ° PREP TIME: 5 MINUTES ° COOK TIME: 10 MINUTES

DAIRY-FREE
NUT-FREE

1 scallion, white and green
parts, thinly sliced

1 teaspoon minced garlic

½ cup gluten-free
bread crumbs

1 egg

2 tablespoons mayonnaise

1 teaspoon Old Bay
Seasoning

1 pound lump crabmeat,
picked over for shells

Sea salt

Freshly ground
black pepper

2 tablespoons extra-virgin
olive oil

Purchased crab cakes should really be called "wheat cakes" for the amount of bread crumbs typically packed into them. This version uses a fraction of the usual amount for an especially "crabby" crab cake.

1. In a medium bowl, combine the scallion, garlic, bread crumbs, egg, mayonnaise, and Old Bay Seasoning. Whisk until thoroughly combined.

2. Fold in the crabmeat, trying not to break up the larger pieces of crab. Season with salt and pepper. Form the crab mixture into 6 individual cakes.

3. Heat a large skillet or sauté pan over medium-high heat until hot. Add the olive oil and tilt the pan to coat the bottom.

4. Cook the crab cakes for 4 to 5 minutes on each side, until they're golden brown.

INGREDIENT TIP If you don't have Old Bay Seasoning, you can use any gluten-free crab boil seasoning you find. Or, make your own by mixing the following ingredients: 1 tablespoon celery salt, 1 tablespoon crumbled bay leaves, 1 teaspoon paprika, ½ teaspoon freshly ground black pepper, ¼ teaspoon dry mustard, ⅛ teaspoon cayenne pepper, 1 pinch ground nutmeg, 1 pinch ground cloves, and 1 pinch ground cinnamon. Makes about 3 tablespoons. Store in an airtight jar in a cool, dark place.

PER SERVING Calories 551; Total Carbohydrates 24g; Sugar 3g; Total Fat 27g; Saturated Fat 4g; Sodium 1084mg; Protein 53g; Fiber 2g

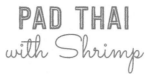

PAD THAI
with Shrimp

SERVES 4 ° PREP TIME: 10 MINUTES ° COOK TIME: 15 MINUTES

DAIRY-FREE

8 ounces flat rice noodles

½ cup hot water, plus more for covering the noodles

½ cup gluten-free fish sauce

¼ cup packed brown sugar

2 tablespoons tamarind concentrate

3 tablespoons canola oil, divided

16 ounces large shrimp, peeled and deveined

4 eggs, whisked

4 scallions, white and green parts, thinly sliced on the bias

2 garlic cloves, minced

¼ teaspoon red pepper flakes

1½ cups mung bean sprouts

½ cup fresh cilantro leaves

½ cup roughly chopped roasted peanuts

2 limes, cut into wedges

Creating pad Thai at home is somewhat like finding the pot of gold at the end of the rainbow—it is both elusive and, the closer you get, the more you lose track of where you're heading. First, what is the essence of pad Thai? For most of us, it's wrapped up in that first time we tried the dish and were undone by the combination of sweet, sour, and umami flavors coalescing in a heap of pasta topped with peanuts. I hope my quick and easy version answers your need for tasty homemade takeout without the gluten.

1. In a large heatproof container, combine the rice noodles with enough hot water to cover them. Soak for 10 minutes and then drain thoroughly.

2. In a medium bowl, combine the ½ cup hot water, fish sauce, brown sugar, and tamarind concentrate. Stir to dissolve the sugar and tamarind concentrate. Set the sauce aside.

3. Heat a large skillet or wok over medium-high heat. Add 1 tablespoon of the canola oil and tilt the pan to coat the bottom.

4. Add the shrimp and fry for about 5 minutes until cooked through. Transfer to a dish.

5. Return the pan to the heat and add 1 tablespoon of the canola oil. When it is hot, add the eggs. Cook in a thin layer on the bottom of the pan for 1 to 2 minutes until set. Fold the egg into an omelet, slice thinly, and transfer to a separate dish.

6. Return the pan to the heat and add the remaining 1 tablespoon canola oil. When hot, add the scallions, garlic, and red pepper flakes. Sauté for about 30 seconds, just until fragrant.

7. Drain the noodles and add them to the pan. Sauté for about 30 seconds until warmed through.

8. Add the sauce to the pan and cook for 2 minutes. (The noodles will absorb some of the sauce.)

9. Add the cooked shrimp and egg to the pan. Toss to combine and cook for about 1 minute, just until heated through.

10. To serve, garnish with the bean sprouts, cilantro, peanuts, and lime wedges.

INGREDIENT TIP Tamarind concentrate is found in most Asian markets and online, but if you cannot find it, opt for tamarind paste or pulp. It is sold in a block wrapped in plastic and will contain the seedpods or skin. Soak ½ cup of the paste in 1 cup of very hot water. Massage it with your fingers to break up the lumps, and then let it rest for 5 minutes before pressing through a fine-mesh sieve.

VARIATION TIP For even more deliciousness and nutrients, consider adding 2 cups of roughly chopped fresh spinach with the scallions, garlic, and red pepper flakes in step 6, and finish the recipe as directed.

PER SERVING Calories 546; Total Carbohydrates 38g; Sugar 15g; Total Fat 26g; Saturated Fat 4g; Sodium 3142mg; Protein 42g; Fiber 3g

SHRIMP BIBIMBAP

SERVES 4 ∘ PREP TIME: 10 MINUTES ∘ COOK TIME: 20 MINUTES

DAIRY-FREE
NUT-FREE

1½ cups white rice
2 cups water
Sea salt
1 teaspoon minced
    peeled fresh ginger
1 teaspoon minced garlic
2 tablespoons gluten-free
    soy sauce, plus more
    for serving
1 tablespoon Sriracha
    chili sauce
1 tablespoon plus
    1 teaspoon toasted
    sesame oil, divided
1 tablespoon freshly
    squeezed lime juice
1 tablespoon honey
1 pound large shrimp,
    peeled and deveined
4 cups fresh spinach
1 cup sliced button
    mushrooms
1 tablespoon canola oil
4 eggs
2 tablespoons toasted
    sesame seeds
1 cup kimchee (optional)

The first time I made this flavorful take on a Korean rice bowl for Rich, he said, "Feel free to put this on the menu every week." It works well for our family because everyone enjoys rice and vegetables, and each person can customize it to suit their preference with shrimp, eggs, and kimchee. For the kids, I cook it as indicated, but when it's just the two of us, I add another tablespoon of Sriracha.

1. In a medium pot over medium-high heat, bring the rice, water, and a generous pinch salt to a simmer. Cover and cook on low for about 20 minutes, until the rice is tender.

2. While the rice cooks, in a small nonreactive bowl, whisk the ginger, garlic, soy sauce, Sriracha, 1 tablespoon of the sesame oil, lime juice, and honey. Let the sauce rest for 5 minutes.

3. In a large skillet or sauté pan over medium heat, cook the shrimp with all of the sauce for about 3 minutes, until cooked through and opaque. Transfer to a clean bowl.

4. Place another large skillet over medium heat. Add the remaining 1 teaspoon sesame oil, the spinach, and mushrooms. Sauté for 3 to 5 minutes until the spinach is soft and most of the moisture has evaporated. Transfer to a clean bowl.

5. Wipe the skillet clean and place it over high heat. Add the canola oil and tilt the pan to coat the bottom. Carefully crack the eggs into the pan and fry for 3 to 5 minutes until set.

6. Evenly divide the cooked rice among 4 serving bowls. Top each with cooked shrimp and spinach, then finish with a fried egg.

7. Sprinkle with sesame seeds, and serve with kimchee (if using) and additional soy sauce.

INGREDIENT TIP Purchase peeled and deveined shrimp from the fish counter to save time. If that is not available, look for easy-peel shrimp.

COOKING TIP This recipe cooks up quickly, so have all the ingredients prepared before you begin.

PER SERVING Calories 586; Total Carbohydrates 67g; Sugar 5g; Total Fat 17g; Saturated Fat 3g; Sodium 904mg; Protein 39g; Fiber 2g

COCONUT-CRUSTED SHRIMP

SERVES 4 ° PREP TIME: 10 MINUTES ° COOK TIME: 5 TO 7 MINUTES

DAIRY-FREE
NUT-FREE

¼ cup Whole-Grain
  Gluten-Free Flour
  Blend (page 25)
1 ½ cups unsweetened
  shredded coconut
2 egg whites
½ teaspoon sea salt
¼ teaspoon garlic powder
1 ½ pounds jumbo shrimp,
  peeled and butterflied
¼ cup coconut oil

Sometimes I long for the crispy, coconut-crusted, succulent shrimp so popular on restaurant appetizer menus. Fortunately, a gluten-free version is easy to make at home, with no unhealthy dip in a deep fryer needed.

1. Place the flour blend in a small bowl.

2. Place the coconut in another small bowl.

3. In a third small bowl, whisk the egg whites, salt, and garlic powder.

4. Dip each shrimp into the flour blend, then the egg white mixture, and then dredge in the coconut. Place each on a plate.

5. Heat a large skillet or sauté pan over medium-high heat until hot, about 2 minutes.

6. Melt the coconut oil in the skillet and tilt the pan to coat the bottom.

7. When the oil is hot, transfer the shrimp to the pan and cook for 2 to 3 minutes on each side until golden brown, crisp, and cooked through.

COOKING TIP To butterfly shrimp, use a paring knife to slice along the back of the peeled shrimp. Devein, if you have not already done so, and fold the shrimp open as if opening a book.

PER SERVING Calories 383; Total Carbohydrates 11g; Sugar 5g; Total Fat 24g; Saturated Fat 21g; Sodium 2231mg; Protein 34g; Fiber 3g

STEAMED MUSSELS

SERVES 4 ° PREP TIME: 10 MINUTES ° COOK TIME: 15 MINUTES

EGG-FREE
NUT-FREE
ONE POT
SPLURGE-WORTHY

2 tablespoons extra-virgin olive oil

3 tablespoons cold butter, divided

1 yellow onion, diced

4 garlic cloves, minced

1 teaspoon fresh thyme leaves

3 pounds fresh mussels, scrubbed and debearded

½ cup dry white wine

Sea salt

Freshly ground black pepper

½ cup roughly chopped fresh parsley

1 lemon, halved

This recipe for steamed mussels is another appetizer menu staple, and rightly so because it's simply delicious. Sop up the juices with a generous chunk of gluten-free bread or serve it over a heap of gluten-free pasta.

1. In a large pot over medium heat, heat the olive oil and melt 1 tablespoon of the butter.

2. Add the onion, garlic, and thyme and cook for about 5 minutes, until the onion is somewhat softened.

3. Add the mussels and white wine and give everything a good toss. Season generously with salt and pepper. Cover and cook until the mussels steam open, about 5 minutes.

4. Transfer any opened mussels to a serving dish, while cooking the rest until all are opened. Discard any mussels that have not opened after 10 minutes.

5. Continue simmering the pan juices for another 2 to 3 minutes until somewhat reduced.

6. Whisk in the remaining 2 tablespoons butter, one tablespoon at a time, to thicken the sauce. Pour the sauce over the mussels.

7. Shower with the fresh parsley and squeeze the lemon juice over, watching for any seeds. Serve immediately.

INGREDIENT TIP Wait until you're ready to cook the mussels to remove the stringy "beards" that emerge from their shells. The mussels are alive until then.

PER SERVING Calories 472; Total Carbohydrates 18g; Sugar 2g; Total Fat 23g; Saturated Fat 8g; Sodium 1100mg; Protein 41g; Fiber 1g

NEW ENGLAND
Clam Chowder

SERVES 4 ° PREP TIME: 15 MINUTES ° COOK TIME: 30 MINUTES

EGG-FREE
NUT-FREE
ONE POT

4 bacon slices, cut
  into small strips
4 Yukon Gold potatoes,
  peeled and diced
3 celery stalks,
  finely diced
1 onion, finely diced
4 garlic cloves, minced
1 teaspoon minced
  fresh thyme
Sea salt
2 tablespoons Whole-
  Grain Gluten-Free
  Flour Blend (page 25)
2 cups whole milk
2 cups low-sodium
  chicken broth
Freshly ground
  black pepper
2 (6-ounce) cans clams,
  drained and roughly
  chopped

Traditional clam chowder in restaurants is often thickened with wheat flour. This gluten-free version is just as delicious and uses my Whole-Grain Gluten-Free Flour Blend (page 25) to thicken it.

1. In a large pot over medium-low heat, cook the bacon for about 8 minutes, stirring frequently, until it renders most of its fat. Use a slotted spoon to transfer the bacon to a separate dish and set aside. Leave the fat in the pot.

2. Add the potatoes, celery, onion, garlic, and thyme to the pot and season with salt. Cook for 5 to 7 minutes while stirring often, until the vegetables soften slightly.

3. Stir in the flour blend and cook for about 2 minutes, until thick and golden brown.

4. Stir in the milk and chicken broth and bring to a gentle simmer. Season with salt and pepper. Cover and cook for 10 minutes until the vegetables are tender.

5. Stir in the clams and cook for about 1 minute more, just until heated through.

6. Ladle the soup into individual serving bowls and garnish with the cooked bacon.

COOKING TIP You can also use fresh clams in this recipe. Add them during the last 5 minutes of cooking time and cook until they are opened. Discard any that do not open.

PER SERVING Calories 448; Total Carbohydrates 53g; Sugar 12g; Total Fat 17g; Saturated Fat 7g; Sodium 1481mg; Protein 22g; Fiber 4g

SEARED SEA SCALLOPS

SERVES 4 ° PREP TIME: 2 MINUTES ° COOK TIME: 12 TO 16 MINUTES

EGG-FREE
NUT-FREE
ONE POT
SPLURGE-WORTHY

2 tablespoons extra-virgin
   olive oil, divided
2 tablespoons
   butter, divided
1 ½ pounds jumbo or
   colossal sea scallops
Sea salt
Freshly ground
   black pepper

Serve these scallops over Creamy Polenta (page 98) for a filling and complete meal. Sea scallops—especially the colossal ones that are good for pan searing—are pricey. Wait until they're in season and on sale at your local market. The recipe is cooked in two batches, so as not to crowd the pan.

1. Heat a large skillet or sauté pan over medium-high heat until hot. Heat 1 tablespoon of the olive oil and melt 1 tablespoon of the butter in the skillet and swirl the pan to coat.

2. Pat half of the scallops dry with a paper towel. Season generously with salt and pepper.

3. When the butter foams and begins to brown, place the seasoned scallops into the pan. Cook for 2 to 3 minutes until a golden-brown crust forms on the bottom, basting continuously with the pan juices.

4. Flip the scallops and cook for 1 minute, basting as you go. Transfer the cooked scallops to a warmed serving dish.

5. Add the remaining 1 tablespoon olive oil and the butter to the skillet. Cook the remaining scallops as in steps 2 and 3. Transfer the cooked scallops to the serving dish and serve immediately.

COOKING TIP To baste the scallops, gently tilt the pan to the side and use a soup spoon to scoop up the butter, oil, and pan juices and pour over each scallop.

PER SERVING Calories 261; Total Carbohydrates 4g; Sugar 0g; Total Fat 14g; Saturated Fat 5g; Sodium 373mg; Protein 29g; Fiber 0g

SPICY GRILLED SHRIMP
and Vegetable Kebabs

SERVES 4 ° PREP TIME: 5 MINUTES ° COOK TIME: 10 MINUTES

DAIRY-FREE
EGG-FREE
NUT-FREE
ONE POT

4 garlic cloves, minced
1 tablespoon
  smoked paprika
½ teaspoon sea salt
⅛ teaspoon
  cayenne pepper
2 tablespoons extra-virgin
  olive oil
Zest of 1 lemon
Juice of 1 lemon
2 pounds jumbo shrimp,
  peeled and deveined
2 medium zucchini, halved
  lengthwise and cut
  into 1-inch pieces
1 pint grape tomatoes
1 red onion, cut into
  1-inch chunks

These shrimp and vegetable kebabs are my summer grilling staple! This recipe can be prepared ahead of time and then chilled and served cold over rice or mixed greens.

1. In a small bowl, mix the garlic, paprika, salt, cayenne pepper, olive oil, lemon zest, and lemon juice.

2. Alternating between the shrimp and vegetables, thread them onto bamboo or wooden skewers and place them in a shallow dish or on a plate.

3. Pour the marinade over the kebabs and let rest for 5 minutes.

4. Heat a gas grill or grill pan to medium heat until the grates are hot, about 5 minutes. Sear the skewers for 3 to 4 minutes on each side, continuously basting with the marinade, until the vegetables are lightly browned and the shrimp are cooked through. Serve immediately.

COOKING TIP Many recipes call for soaking wooden skewers in water ahead of time to prevent them from burning. I do not recommend this because it makes the inside of the food soggy and I have yet to light a skewer on fire.

PER SERVING Calories 382; Total Carbohydrates 15g; Sugar 6g; Total Fat 12g; Saturated Fat 2g; Sodium 804mg; Protein 54g; Fiber 4g

CHILE LIME COD

SERVES 4 ° PREP TIME: 5 MINUTES ° COOK TIME: 15 MINUTES

DAIRY-FREE
EGG-FREE
NUT-FREE

4 (6-ounce) cod fillets
Juice of 1 lime
Zest of 1 lime
1 tablespoon ancho
  chile powder
1 teaspoon
  smoked paprika
1 teaspoon ground
  coriander
½ teaspoon sea salt
¼ teaspoon freshly
  ground black pepper
⅛ teaspoon
  cayenne pepper
2 tablespoons canola oil

Ancho chile powder and smoked paprika form a delicious crust around tender cod. Use another somewhat firm, flaky white fish if you don't like cod. Serve this with steamed rice or the Avocado, Black Bean, and Quinoa Salad (page 95).

1. Pat the cod fillets dry with a paper towel and put on a plate. Sprinkle each fillet evenly with the lime juice.

2. In a shallow dish, mix the lime zest, ancho chile powder, paprika, coriander, salt, black pepper, and cayenne pepper.

3. Coat the cod fillets with the spice mixture.

4. In a large skillet or sauté pan over medium-high heat, heat the canola oil until hot.

5. Sear the fish for 3 to 4 minutes on each side, or until cooked through and the fish flakes easily with a fork.

INGREDIENT TIP Frozen fish is often fresher than what you purchase at the fish counter, which is often frozen and thawed perhaps a day or two before you purchase it.

PER SERVING Calories 242; Total Carbohydrates 0g; Sugar 0g; Total Fat 9g; Saturated Fat 1g; Sodium 367mg; Protein 39g; Fiber 0g

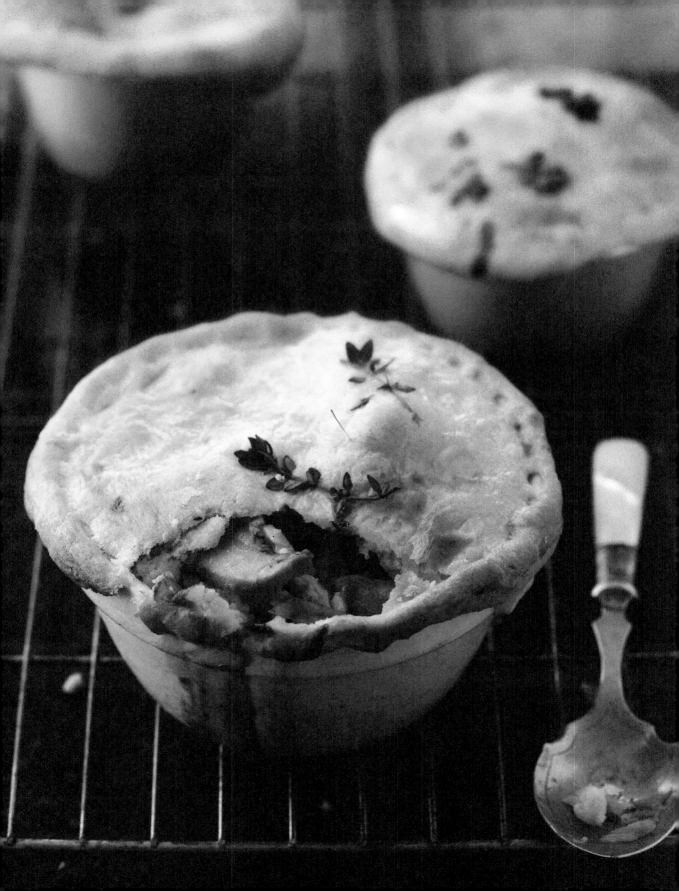

CHAPTER Six

MEAT AND POULTRY

PAN-SEARED CHICKEN BREAST
with Sautéed Zucchini

SERVES 4 ∘ PREP TIME: 5 MINUTES ∘ COOK TIME: 20 MINUTES

ALLERGEN-FREE
DAIRY-FREE
EGG-FREE
NUT-FREE
ONE POT

2 to 3 tablespoons extra-
 virgin olive oil, divided
3 to 4 (4- to 6-ounce)
 boneless skinless chicken
 breasts, pounded to a
 uniform ½-inch thickness
Sea salt
Freshly ground
 black pepper
2 medium zucchini,
 quartered lengthwise,
 cut into ½-inch pieces
½ cup dry red wine,
 such as Merlot

This is the kind of dish I could order in a restaurant and be completely satisfied. It is also the kind of recipe I wouldn't give a second look if I saw it in a cookbook. With just a handful of ingredients, how could it be good, let alone epic? It's all about technique—specifically high heat and liberal seasoning. The red wine sauce seems like an afterthought, but it's totally worth it. Serve with Sour Cream Mashed Potatoes (page 96).

1. Heat a large skillet or sauté pan over medium-high heat until hot, about 2 minutes. Add 1 tablespoon of the olive oil to the pan and tilt the pan to coat the bottom.

2. Pat the chicken breasts dry with paper towels and liberally season both sides with salt and pepper. Place in the skillet and cook for 5 minutes until well browned. Flip and cook for 4 to 5 minutes on the other side until cooked through. Transfer to serving plates.

3. Return the skillet to medium-high heat and add another 1 tablespoon olive oil to the pan.

4. Add the zucchini and sauté for about 3 minutes, until browned on the outside but still somewhat firm. Season with salt and pepper, and transfer to the serving plates.

5. Carefully add the red wine to the pan. Simmer for about 2 minutes, stirring frequently, until reduced to a few tablespoons.

6. Drizzle in 1 to 2 teaspoons of the remaining olive oil and whisk to combine. Pour the sauce over the chicken and zucchini and serve.

SERVING TIP The recipe calls for 3 or 4 chicken breasts. If you're serving this to young children, they will likely split one breast. Also, although most of the alcohol cooks off, I leave the red wine sauce off my kids' plates.

PER SERVING Calories 453; Total Carbohydrates 4g; Sugar 2g; Total Fat 23g; Saturated Fat 5g; Sodium 216g; Protein 50g; Fiber 1g

GARLIC HONEY CHICKEN
and Vegetables

SERVES 4 ∘ PREP TIME: 10 MINUTES ∘ COOK TIME: 15 MINUTES

ALLERGEN-FREE
DAIRY-FREE
EGG-FREE
NUT-FREE
ONE POT

2 tablespoons extra-virgin
 olive oil, divided
4 (4- to 6-ounce) boneless
 skinless chicken breasts,
 pounded to a uniform
 ½-inch thickness
Sea salt
Freshly ground
 black pepper
1 head broccoli, cut
 into small florets
2 carrots, cut into
 narrow strips
2 teaspoons minced garlic
1 teaspoon minced
 fresh thyme
1 tablespoon honey
1 teaspoon Dijon mustard
2 tablespoons plus
 1 teaspoon freshly
 squeezed lemon juice

Sweet honey, aromatic garlic, and tangy lemon juice marry beautifully in this simple panfried chicken recipe. Don't be surprised when everyone asks for seconds!

1. Heat a large skillet or sauté pan over medium-high heat until hot, about 2 minutes. Add 1 tablespoon of the olive oil to the pan and tilt the pan to coat the bottom.

2. Pat the chicken breasts dry with paper towels and liberally season both sides with salt and pepper. Place in the skillet and cook for 5 minutes until well browned. Flip and cook for 4 to 5 minutes on the other side until cooked through. Transfer to serving plates.

3. Add the remaining tablespoon olive oil to the pan. Add the broccoli and carrots and sauté for about 4 minutes until crisp-tender. Season with salt and pepper. Transfer to the serving plates.

4. Reduce the heat to medium-low. Add the garlic and thyme to the pan and cook for 30 seconds.

5. In a glass liquid measuring cup, whisk the honey, mustard, and 2 tablespoons of the lemon juice and pour into the pan, stirring to scrape up any browned bits from the bottom of the pan.

6. Drizzle the sauce over the chicken, sprinkle the vegetables with the remaining 1 teaspoon lemon juice, and serve.

INGREDIENT TIP This recipe is also really good with bone-in skin-on chicken thighs. Increase the cooking time to about 10 minutes on each side for the chicken, and use a thermometer to ensure it reaches an internal temperature of 165°F.

PER SERVING Calories 440; Total Carbohydrates 13g; Sugar 7g; Total Fat 20g; Saturated Fat 5g; Sodium 264mg; Protein 53g; Fiber 3g

SPICY SWEET POTATO
Chicken Soup

SERVES 4 ○ PREP TIME: 5 MINUTES ○ COOK TIME: 25 MINUTES

EGG-FREE
NUT-FREE
ONE POT
MAKE ALLERGEN-FREE
MAKE DAIRY-FREE

1 tablespoon extra-virgin
olive oil
1 onion, diced
3 garlic cloves, minced
1 quart gluten-free
chicken broth, or Chicken
Stock (page 212)
2 cups peeled, diced
sweet potatoes
1 roasted red bell pepper,
cut into thin strips
1 cup fire-roasted
corn kernels
1 cup salsa verde
1 teaspoon ground cumin
1 teaspoon smoked paprika
Pinch cayenne pepper
2 (4- to 6-ounce) boneless
skinless chicken breasts
Sea salt
Freshly ground
black pepper
1 teaspoon freshly
squeezed lime juice
8 ounces sour cream
(optional)
½ cup roughly chopped
fresh cilantro

This spicy soup is perfect any time of the year, but I especially love it in the fall when the leaves begin to turn and you just want something warm. But it's also good on blazing-hot summer days—the spiciness of the soup matches the intensity of the weather.

1. In a large pot over medium heat, heat the olive oil.

2. Add the onion and garlic and cook, stirring frequently, for about 5 minutes until soft.

3. Add the chicken broth, sweet potatoes, bell pepper, corn, salsa verde, cumin, paprika, cayenne pepper, and chicken breasts. Season with salt and pepper and stir to combine.

4. Bring to a simmer, cover, and cook for 20 minutes until the sweet potatoes are tender and the chicken is cooked through.

5. Remove the chicken from the soup and shred it with two forks. Return the shredded meat to the soup and stir in the lime juice.

6. Ladle the soup into a serving bowl and top with the sour cream (if using) and the cilantro. Serve with gluten-free tortilla chips or corn chips on the side, if desired.

SUBSTITUTION TIP To make this dairy-free and allergen-free, omit the sour cream.

PER SERVING Calories 632; Total Carbohydrates 59g; Sugar 7g; Total Fat 32g; Saturated Fat 11g; Sodium 1500mg; Protein 33g; Fiber 8g

COCONUT MILK AND
Thyme Poached Chicken

SERVES 4 ° PREP TIME: 5 MINUTES ° COOK TIME: 20 TO 25 MINUTES

DAIRY-FREE
EGG-FREE
NUT-FREE
ONE POT
SLOW COOKER OPTION

1 tablespoon extra-virgin
   olive oil
6 to 8 (4- to 6-ounce)
   bone-in skinless
   chicken thighs
Sea salt
Freshly ground
   black pepper
1 shallot, minced
4 garlic cloves, crushed
1 tablespoon fresh
   thyme leaves
1 cup full-fat coconut milk
1 cup gluten-free chicken
   broth, or Chicken
   Stock (page 212)
2 cups green beans,
   stemmed

I adore poached chicken because it is so tender and moist, especially when you use bone-in pieces of meat.

1. In a large skillet or sauté pan over medium-high heat, heat the olive oil.

2. Pat the chicken thighs dry with a paper towel and generously season both sides with salt and pepper. Place them top-side down (where the skin was) into the skillet to brown. Cook for 5 minutes. Flip the chicken and cook for 4 minutes more.

3. Add the shallot, garlic, and thyme to the pan. Cook for 30 seconds.

4. Stir in the coconut milk and chicken broth, scraping up any browned bits from the bottom of the pan.

5. Add the green beans. Reduce the heat to medium-low, cover, and cook for 10 to 15 minutes, or until the chicken is cooked through and the green beans are tender.

6. Serve in shallow bowls.

SLOW COOKER OPTION Place all ingredients into the slow cooker, cover, and cook for 8 hours on low.

SERVING TIP Serve with steamed rice or a crusty gluten-free baguette.

PER SERVING Calories 627; Total Carbohydrates 9g; Sugar 3g; Total Fat 35g; Saturated Fat 18g; Sodium 458mg; Protein 69g; Fiber 4g

BASIC ROAST CHICKEN

SERVES 4 TO 6 ∘ PREP TIME: 5 MINUTES ∘ COOK TIME: 25 MINUTES

DAIRY-FREE
EGG-FREE
NUT-FREE
ONE POT

1 (4-pound) whole chicken
1 tablespoon extra-virgin
  olive oil
Sea salt
Freshly ground
  black pepper

The only way to cook a chicken in 30 minutes happens to be one of the most flavorful ways: spatchcock. It involves splitting the bird open so the inside of the chicken faces the pan. This technique allows the skin to become deliciously crisp and the meat to cook evenly. It takes a little bit of chutzpah and elbow grease to remove the backbone, but you've got this!

1. Preheat the oven to 425°F.

2. Working in a clean sink, stand the chicken on one end, with the breasts facing away from you and the backbone in front of you. Firmly grasp one end of the backbone in one hand. Using a sharp knife or a pair of kitchen shears, cut down one side of the backbone. Be careful to keep your hand away from the blade.

3. Turn the chicken upside down (so you can continue to use your dominant hand) and slice down the other side of the backbone. Remove it and reserve it for another use, such as making Chicken Stock (page 212).

4. Place the chicken on a rimmed baking sheet, cut-side down, and spread out the legs. Press down on the breasts with the heel of your hand so the chicken lies flat.

5. Pat the chicken dry with paper towels and coat it with olive oil. Generously season both sides with salt and pepper.

6. Roast uncovered for 25 minutes, or until the juices run clear and the chicken reaches an internal temperature of 165°F. Smaller birds will cook more quickly. Larger birds will take additional time. Let the chicken rest for at least 5 minutes before serving.

INGREDIENT TIP Purchasing a whole chicken usually saves money. It is often half the cost of prepared cuts of meat.

SERVING TIP In my house, we take turns for who gets the legs and who gets the breast meat. We always have leftovers, which make a perfect addition to lunch salads and burritos.

PER SERVING Calories 174; Total Carbohydrates 3g; Sugar 1g; Total Fat 6g; Saturated Fat 1g; Sodium 322mg; Protein 25g; Fiber 0g

INDIVIDUAL CHICKEN POTPIES

SERVES 4 ° PREP TIME: 1O MINUTES ° COOK TIME: 2O MINUTES

5 tablespoons
 butter, divided
1 cup mushrooms
1 ¼ cups plus
 2 tablespoons Whole-
 Grain Gluten-Free Flour
 Blend (page 25)
½ cup gluten-free chicken
 broth, or Chicken
 Stock (page 212)
2 cups shredded
 cooked chicken
2 cups frozen
 diced carrots
2 cups frozen peas
4 Yukon Gold potatoes,
 peeled and diced
½ teaspoon sea salt
⅓ cup shortening
1 egg
1 to 2 teaspoons ice water
Fresh thyme sprigs,
 for garnish

This recipe is a huge hit with families; kids love to get their very own potpie to eat. Plus, this is a great way to use up leftover chicken meat from the Basic Roast Chicken (page 128). Use the backbone and chicken carcass to make Chicken Stock (page 212) or use a gluten-free prepared chicken broth if you're short on time.

1. Preheat the oven to 425°F.

2. Coat the inside of four 16-ounce, oven-safe ramekins with 1 tablespoon of butter (divided between them).

3. In a large skillet or sauté pan over medium heat, melt 2 tablespoons of the butter. Add the mushrooms and sauté until soft, about 5 minutes. Set aside.

4. In another large skillet over medium heat, melt the remaining 2 tablespoons butter. Whisk in 2 tablespoons of gluten-free flour blend and cook for 1 to 2 minutes. Pour in the chicken broth and stir until thickened.

5. Add the chicken, carrots, peas, and potatoes. Bring to a simmer and cook for about 5 minutes.

6. In a food processor, combine the remaining 1¼ cups flour blend, butter, salt, shortening, and egg. Pulse a few times, just until integrated. Add 1 to 2 teaspoons ice water to bind the crust mixture. With a rolling pin, roll the crust between two sheets of parchment paper to about ¼-inch thickness. Remove the top sheet of parchment paper.

7. Invert one of the ramekins onto the pastry dough and trace around it with a knife, cutting both the dough and the parchment paper underneath. Repeat until all four pastry circles are cut.

8. Transfer the chicken and vegetable mixture into the prepared ramekins, and invert each pastry circle onto the chicken and vegetables. Carefully peel away the second sheet of parchment. Press the sides of the crusts onto the ramekin edges to seal, cutting away or folding under any excess.

9. Bake for 20 minutes, or until the tops are golden brown and the filling is bubbling. Garnish with fresh thyme sprigs and serve.

COOKING TIP If you have difficulty removing the parchment paper from the crusts, place the crusts in the freezer for up to 5 minutes.

PER SERVING Calories 764; Total Carbohydrates 78g; Sugar 8g; Total Fat 36g; Saturated Fat 15g; Sodium 606mg; Protein 35g; Fiber 9g

PANFRIED CRISPY CHICKEN

SERVES 4 ° PREP TIME: 5 MINUTES ° COOK TIME: 25 MINUTES

NUT-FREE
ONE POT

1 cup buttermilk
1 egg, whisked
6 to 8 (4- to 6-ounce)
  bone-in skin-on
  chicken thighs
1 cup Whole-Grain
  Gluten-Free Flour
  Blend (page 25)
1 tablespoon paprika
1 teaspoon garlic powder
1 teaspoon onion powder
1 teaspoon sea salt
1 teaspoon freshly ground
  black pepper
¼ cup canola oil

During my first few months of marriage, I set my apartment kitchen on fire making tempura—deep-fried shrimp and vegetables. Thirteen years later, I'm still skittish about using a deep fryer, especially with two rambunctious boys running around. That said, I miss the crispy skin of deep-fried chicken. Here's the gluten-free answer to my longing.

1. Preheat the oven to 425°F.

2. In a large nonreactive dish, whisk the buttermilk and egg. Add the chicken and turn to coat. Set aside.

3. In a separate dish, combine the flour blend, paprika, garlic powder, onion powder, salt, and pepper. Set aside.

4. Heat a large cast-iron skillet over medium-high heat. Add the canola oil to the pan and heat until hot but not smoking.

5. Working one piece at a time, remove the chicken from the buttermilk and shake off any excess. Dredge it in the flour mixture, shake off any excess, and then place it into the skillet, skin-side down. Repeat with the remaining chicken thighs. Cook for 5 minutes, flip the chicken, and transfer the skillet to the oven.

6. Continue cooking for 20 minutes, or until the chicken is cooked through and the skin is crisp. Serve hot.

COOKING TIP Here's how to tell if the oil is hot enough. Sprinkle the tiniest bit of flour into the oil. If it floats away, the oil is hot.

PER SERVING Calories 716; Total Carbohydrates 29g; Sugar 4g; Total Fat 33g; Saturated Fat 6g; Sodium 745mg; Protein 73g; Fiber 2g

PROVENÇAL CHICKEN STEW

SERVES 4 ° PREP TIME: 5 MINUTES ° COOK TIME: 25 MINUTES

DAIRY-FREE
EGG-FREE
NUT-FREE
ONE POT
SLOW COOKER OPTION

1 tablespoon extra-virgin
  olive oil
4 to 6 (4- to 6-ounce)
  bone-in skinless
  chicken thighs
Sea salt
Freshly ground
  black pepper
4 new potatoes, scrubbed
  and quartered
4 carrots, unpeeled,
  cut into 2-inch pieces
2 shallots, quartered
  lengthwise
2 teaspoons herbes
  de Provence
4 garlic cloves, smashed
½ cup dry white wine
1 (15-ounce) can whole
  plum tomatoes, drained
2 cups gluten-free chicken
  broth, or Chicken
  Stock (page 212)

This healthy chicken stew is very easy to throw together, and the flavors are truly classic and comforting. It's perfect for a rich, filling dinner or hearty lunch on a busy day.

1. In a large pot over medium-high heat, heat the olive oil.

2. Pat the chicken thighs dry with a paper towel and generously season both sides with salt and pepper.

3. Place the chicken top-side down (where the skin was) into the pot and sear for 3 to 4 minutes. Flip the chicken and add the potatoes, carrots, shallots, herbes de Provence, and garlic.

4. Pour in the white wine, deglazing the pan by scraping up any browned bits from the bottom.

5. Add the tomatoes and chicken broth. Bring to a simmer, cover, reduce the heat to low, and cook for 20 minutes, or until the chicken is cooked through and the potatoes are tender.

INGREDIENT TIP If you do not have dried herbes de Provence, you can make your own by combining equal parts thyme, rosemary, marjoram, and oregano. A little lavender is also a lovely addition. Store extra in a sealed jar in a dark place.

SLOW COOKER OPTION To make in a slow cooker, skip browning the thighs and cook on low for 8 hours until the chicken is cooked through.

PER SERVING Calories 432; Total Carbohydrates 22g; Sugar 7g; Total Fat 15g; Saturated Fat 4g; Sodium 615g; Protein 46g; Fiber 4g

CHICKEN AND SAUSAGE
with Wine Reduction

SERVES 4 ∘ PREP TIME: 5 MINUTES ∘ COOK TIME: 20 MINUTES

1½ tablespoons plus
  2 teaspoons extra-virgin
  olive oil, divided
3 to 4 (4- to 6-ounce)
  boneless skinless chicken
  breasts, pounded to a
  uniform ½-inch thickness
Sea salt
Freshly ground
  black pepper
2 gluten-free Italian
  sausages, casings
  removed
Sour Cream Mashed
  Potatoes (optional,
  page 96)
1 cup dry red wine
1 cup low-sodium chicken
  broth, or Chicken
  Stock (page 212)
2 cups fresh arugula
½ lime

One day Rich was out of town and I was on a meat kick. I had some leftover Italian sausage to use and frozen chicken breasts. I made up this recipe and it was so delicious. The meal came together so quickly, I knew I had to share it. It is even more delicious over Sour Cream Mashed Potatoes (page 96).

1. Heat a large skillet or sauté pan over medium-high heat until hot, about 2 minutes. Add 1½ tablespoons of the olive oil to the pan.

2. Pat the chicken breasts dry with paper towels. Liberally season both sides with salt and pepper. Place them in the skillet and cook for 5 minutes until well browned. Flip the chicken breasts and add the sausage to the pan, crumbling it with the back of a spoon. Cook for 4 to 5 minutes more until cooked through.

3. Transfer the chicken and sausage to shallow serving bowls on top of the Sour Cream Mashed Potatoes (if using). Return the skillet to medium-high heat.

4. Carefully add the red wine and chicken broth to the pan. Bring to a simmer and cook for about 4 minutes until reduced to about ⅓ cup. Drizzle in 1 or 2 teaspoons of the remaining olive oil and whisk to combine.

5. Evenly divide the arugula among the serving bowls and sprinkle with lime juice.

6. Pour the wine reduction over the chicken, sausage, and mashed potatoes (if using).

SERVING TIP Use sweet Italian sausage for young palates. Otherwise, spicy Italian sausage is fantastic in this recipe.

PER SERVING Calories 665; Total Carbohydrates 3g; Sugar 1g; Total Fat 41g; Saturated Fat 11g; Sodium 814g; Protein 59g; Fiber 1g

CHICKEN PIZZA ALFREDO

SERVES 2 • PREP TIME: 5 MINUTES PLUS 10 MINUTES INACTIVE TIME
COOK TIME: 15 MINUTES

SPLURGE-WORTHY

FOR THE CRUST
1½ teaspoons sugar
⅓ cup hot water (<110°F)
1 package (2¼ teaspoons)
  active dry yeast
1 cup finely ground
  blanched almond flour
¾ cup tapioca flour (starch)
¾ teaspoon sea salt
1 egg white
1½ teaspoons red
  wine vinegar
¼ cup potato starch
1 to 2 tablespoons extra-
  virgin olive oil

FOR THE TOPPINGS
1 tablespoon mashed
  roasted garlic
1½ cups Cheese Sauce
  (White Sauce, Variation
  Tip with cheese,
  page 214)
2 cups shredded cooked
  chicken breast, from
  the Basic Roast
  Chicken (page 128)
1 teaspoon minced
  fresh thyme
1 cup shredded Italian
  cheese blend

Think of this as your favorite fettucine Alfredo in pizza form. You get the creamy flavor of the sauce with a hearty pizza crust to sop it up. The recipe calls for roasted garlic paste, but it's even better with the cloves from an entire head of garlic, roasted, and then scattered on the pizza.

1. Preheat the oven to 425°F.

2. Place a pizza stone or pizza pan into the oven to heat.

TO MAKE THE CRUST

1. In a small bowl, stir together the sugar and hot water to dissolve the sugar. Add the yeast and whisk with a fork to disburse the yeast granules. Set aside.

2. In a medium bowl, mix the almond flour, tapioca flour, and salt. Make a well in the center of the ingredients. Add the egg white and vinegar.

3. The yeast should be foamy by now. Pour it into the flour mixture and stir to combine. The dough will be quite wet.

4. Add the potato starch and stir to mix thoroughly. Turn the dough out onto a large sheet of parchment paper and spread it into a small circle with a spatula. It will be much wetter than traditional pizza dough.

INGREDIENT TIP Italian cheese blend is usually mozzarella, Romano, Parmesan, and provolone cheeses, but any similar mixture will do.

5. Pour the olive oil onto the pizza dough and your clean hands. Press the dough into a 12-inch circle with your hands. Use your palms to press the center of the dough down and gently nudge the sides of the dough to be somewhat thicker. Let the dough rest for 10 minutes.

6. Slide the pizza dough and parchment paper onto the preheated pizza stone. Bake for 7 minutes.

TO MAKE THE TOPPINGS

1. In a medium bowl, whisk the roasted garlic and cheese sauce.

2. Remove the pizza from the oven; leave the oven on. Top with the cheese sauce, chicken, and thyme.

3. Sprinkle with the cheese blend.

4. Return the pizza to the oven for 8 minutes more until the cheese is browned and bubbling.

COOKING TIP Use bottled roasted garlic or roast your own. Preheat the oven to 400°F. Place a whole head of garlic on a sheet of aluminum foil, drizzle with 1 teaspoon of olive oil, fold the foil into a loose package, and roast for 45 minutes. Squeeze out the garlic cloves and mash into a paste. Alternatively, scatter the whole roasted garlic cloves onto the pizza instead of mashing into a paste.

PER SERVING Calories 1069; Total Carbohydrates 48g; Sugar 6g; Total Fat 60g; Saturated Fat 21g; Sodium 1586mg; Protein 87g; Fiber 5g

SPICY SAUSAGE AND
Caramelized Onion Pizza

SERVES 2 ∘ PREP TIME: 5 MINUTES PLUS 10 MINUTES INACTIVE TIME
COOK TIME: 15 MINUTES

MAKE DAIRY-FREE

FOR THE CRUST
1 ½ teaspoons sugar
⅓ cup hot water (<110°F)
1 package (2 ¼ teaspoons)
   active dry yeast
1 cup finely ground
   blanched almond flour
¾ cup tapioca flour (starch)
¾ teaspoon sea salt
1 egg white
1 ½ teaspoons red wine
   vinegar
¼ cup potato starch
1 to 2 tablespoons extra-
   virgin olive oil

FOR THE TOPPINGS
1 link gluten-free hot
   Italian sausage
1 tablespoon extra-virgin
   olive oil
1 yellow onion, very
   thinly sliced
4 Medjool dates, pitted
   and thinly sliced
½ cup sliced fontina
   cheese (optional)
½ cup fresh basil leaves

While my kids enjoy a plain cheese pizza and Rich opts for the Loaded Vegetarian Pizza (page 162), this is my go-to version. I have to say, this crust makes the best gluten-free pizza I have ever had.

1. Preheat the oven to 425°F.

2. Place a pizza stone or pizza pan in the oven to heat.

TO MAKE THE CRUST

1. In a small bowl, stir together the sugar and hot water to dissolve the sugar. Add the yeast to the water and whisk with a fork to disburse the yeast granules. Set aside.

2. In a medium bowl, mix the almond flour, tapioca flour, and salt. Make a well in the center of the ingredients. Add the egg white and vinegar.

3. The yeast should be foamy by now. Pour it into the mixing bowl and stir to combine. The dough will be quite wet.

4. Add the potato starch and stir to mix thoroughly. Turn out the dough onto a large sheet of parchment paper and spread it into a small circle with a spatula. It will be much wetter than traditional pizza dough.

5. Pour the olive oil onto the pizza dough and your clean hands. Press the dough into a 12-inch circle with your hands. Use your palms to press the center of the dough down and gently nudge the sides of the dough to be somewhat thicker.

6. Set the dough aside to rest for 10 minutes and begin making the toppings.

TO MAKE THE TOPPINGS

1. While the dough rests, place a large skillet or sauté pan over medium heat. Remove the Italian sausage casing, crumble the meat into the pan, and cook for about 5 minutes until browned. Transfer to a separate dish. Add the olive oil and onion to the skillet to cook.

2. Return to the dough. Slide the pizza dough and parchment paper onto the preheated pizza stone. Bake for 10 minutes.

3. Return to the skillet and cook the onions for about 15 minutes, stirring frequently, until browned and soft.

4. Remove the crust from the oven; leave the oven on. Top with the sausage, onions, dates, and fontina cheese (if using).

5. Return the pizza to the oven for 5 minutes more until the cheese is softened.

6. Top with the fresh basil leaves and serve.

COOKING TIP This pizza crust also makes an amazing flatbread. I let it rise for about an hour and top with puréed roasted garlic, minced fresh parsley, and olive oil.

PER SERVING Calories 578; Total Carbohydrates 61g; Sugar 18g; Total Fat 35g; Saturated Fat 5g; Sodium 773g; Protein 11g; Fiber 7g

MOO SHU PORK

SERVES 4 ° PREP TIME: 10 MINUTES ° COOK TIME: 10 MINUTES

DAIRY-FREE
NUT-FREE
ONE POT

¼ cup gluten-free
 hoisin sauce or
 plum sauce
2 tablespoons freshly
 squeezed lime juice
2 tablespoons gluten-free
 soy sauce
1 tablespoon toasted
 sesame oil
1 tablespoon canola oil
2 eggs, whisked
1 pound pork butt,
 thinly sliced
1 tablespoon minced
 peeled fresh ginger
1 teaspoon minced garlic
Pinch red pepper flakes
2 cups shredded red
 cabbage, divided
4 scallions, white and
 green parts, thinly sliced
1 cup thinly sliced shiitake
 mushrooms
Sea salt
Freshly ground
 black pepper
1 head butter lettuce,
 leaves separated

Serve this recipe alongside Stir-Fried Beef and Broccoli (page 143) and steamed rice for a complete dinner with plenty of leftovers. My version of this Chinese restaurant favorite adds Southeast Asian flavors. I also use lettuce wraps instead of a wheat pancake for a lighter and totally gluten-free dish that still tastes amazing.

1. In a sealable jar, combine the hoisin sauce or plum sauce, lime juice, and soy sauce. Seal the lid and shake vigorously to mix the ingredients. Set aside.

2. In a large skillet or sauté pan over medium-high heat, heat the sesame oil and canola oil. Pour in the eggs and cook for about 2 minutes, without disturbing, until set. Fold the omelet in half, and in half again to make a triangle. Transfer to a cutting board to rest.

3. Add the pork to the pan and sauté for 3 to 5 minutes.

4. Add the ginger, garlic, and red pepper flakes. Cook for about 1 minute until fragrant.

5. Add the cabbage, scallions, and mushrooms. Cook for 1 minute.

6. Pour in the sauce and simmer for 1 minute.

7. Thinly slice the egg and fold it into the pork mixture. Season with salt and pepper.

8. Serve with lettuce leaves.

PER SERVING Calories 401; Total Carbohydrates 20g; Sugar 8g; Total Fat 18g; Saturated Fat 4g; Sodium 963mg; Protein 41g; Fiber 3g

PORK MARSALA

SERVES 4 ° PREP TIME: 12 MINUTES ° COOK TIME: 21 MINUTES

EGG-FREE
NUT-FREE
ONE POT

1 tablespoon extra-virgin
  olive oil
2 tablespoons
  butter, divided
4 (5-ounce) boneless pork
  loin chops, pounded to
  about ½-inch thickness
Sea salt
Freshly ground
  black pepper
2 tablespoons Whole-
  Grain Gluten-Free Flour
  Blend (page 25)
2 cups sliced mushrooms
1 shallot, minced
1 garlic clove, minced
1 teaspoon fresh
  thyme leaves
½ cup marsala wine
½ cup gluten-free chicken
  broth, or Chicken
  Stock (page 212)

Most pork marsala prepared in restaurants is coated with wheat flour to produce a delicate crust and thicken the wine sauce. Fortunately, a gluten-free flour blend can do both of these things.

1. In a large skillet or sauté pan over medium-high heat, heat the olive oil and 1 tablespoon of the butter until hot but not smoking.

2. Pat the chops dry with a paper towel and generously season both sides with salt and pepper. Lightly sprinkle the chops on both sides with the flour blend, shaking off any excess. Place the chops in the skillet. Cook for 3 minutes on each side. The pork will not be cooked through. Remove from the skillet and set aside.

3. Add the remaining 1 tablespoon butter to the skillet along with the mushrooms. Sauté for about 4 minutes until browned.

4. Add the shallot, garlic, and thyme to the pan and cook for 30 seconds.

5. Stir in the marsala and deglaze the pan by scraping up any browned bits from the bottom.

6. Add the chicken broth and bring to a simmer. Return the chops to the pan, cover, and cook for 10 minutes.

SERVING TIP Serve this flavorful dish with bright, blanched vegetables, such as green beans, or a simple side salad.

PER SERVING Calories 590; Total Carbohydrates 6g; Sugar 1g; Total Fat 45g; Saturated Fat 17g; Sodium 298mg; Protein 34g; Fiber 1g

PAN-ROASTED PORK CHOPS
with Apples and Potatoes

SERVES 4 ° PREP TIME: 5 MINUTES ° COOK TIME: 25 MINUTES

ALLERGEN-FREE
DAIRY-FREE
EGG-FREE
NUT-FREE
ONE POT

2 tablespoons extra-virgin
  olive oil
4 (6- to 8-ounce) bone-in
  pork chops
Sea salt
Freshly ground
  black pepper
2 Golden Delicious apples,
  peeled, cored, and cut
  into wedges
4 Yukon Gold potatoes,
  quartered
1 teaspoon minced
  fresh thyme

Fruit and pork are meant for each other, especially in this hearty one-pot supper. Excluding salt and pepper, the recipe has only four ingredients, so preparation is a breeze. If you have the time, prepare a simple brine (see Cooking Tip) to keep the pork chops especially moist and juicy through the cooking process.

1. Preheat the oven to 350°F.

2. In a Dutch oven or large cast-iron skillet over medium-high heat, heat 1 tablespoon of the olive oil until very hot.

3. Pat the pork chops dry with a paper towel and season both sides with salt and pepper. Place the chops into the skillet and sear for 3 to 5 minutes to get a golden crust. Flip the pork chops and arrange the apples and potatoes around them. Drizzle with the remaining 1 tablespoon olive oil, sprinkle with the thyme, and season again with salt and pepper.

4. Bake for 20 minutes, or until the pork is cooked to an internal temperature of 145°F and the apples and potatoes are tender.

COOKING TIP To brine the pork chops, dissolve ¼ cup packed brown sugar and ¼ cup sea salt in 1 cup of hot water. Stir to dissolve. Add 2 cups of ice-cold water and pour the mixture over the pork in a nonreactive baking dish. Let rest for 30 minutes before cooking.

PER SERVING Calories 690; Total Carbohydrates 43g; Sugar 11g; Total Fat 43g; Saturated Fat 14g; Sodium 176mg; Protein 36g; Fiber 5g

STIR-FRIED
Beef and Broccoli

SERVES 4 ° PREP TIME: 5 MINUTES ° COOK TIME: 20 MINUTES

2 tablespoons gluten-free soy sauce

1 tablespoon freshly squeezed lime juice

⅛ teaspoon Chinese five-spice powder

1 teaspoon cornstarch

2 tablespoons canola oil, divided

1 pound boneless rib-eye steak

Sea salt

Freshly ground black pepper

1 head broccoli, cut into florets (about 6 cups total)

1 tablespoon minced garlic

1 teaspoon minced peeled fresh ginger

⅛ teaspoon red pepper flakes (optional)

Skip the pricey takeout that's sure to contain gluten and make your own at home. This riff on the classic beef and broccoli on Chinese restaurant menus goes well with steamed rice. Or leave it low-carb and skip the rice. For little ones, omit the red pepper flakes.

1. In a small sealable jar, combine the soy sauce, lime juice, five-spice powder, and cornstarch. Seal the lid and shake vigorously to combine the sauce ingredients.

2. Heat a large cast-iron skillet or wok over medium-high heat. Add 1 tablespoon of the canola oil.

3. Pat the steak dry with paper towels and season both sides with salt and pepper. Put the steak in the hot skillet and cook for 5 to 6 minutes on each side for medium-rare. Transfer the cooked steak to a cutting board.

4. In the same skillet, add the remaining 1 tablespoon canola oil and the broccoli. Sauté for 5 minutes until the broccoli is bright green and crisp-tender.

5. Stir in the garlic, ginger, and red pepper flakes (if using) and cook for 30 seconds.

6. Slice the steak very thinly on a bias and add it, along with any accumulated juices, to the skillet.

7. Pour the sauce into the pan and cook for about 1 minute until it thickens and coats the broccoli and beef.

PER SERVING Calories 346; Total Carbohydrates 11g; Sugar 3g; Total Fat 13g; Saturated Fat 3g; Sodium 606mg; Protein 46g; Fiber 4g

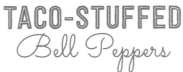

TACO-STUFFED
Bell Peppers

SERVES 4 ° PREP TIME: 10 MINUTES ° COOK TIME: 30 MINUTES

EGG-FREE
NUT-FREE
MAKE ALLERGEN-FREE
MAKE DAIRY-FREE

1 tablespoon extra-virgin
   olive oil
¼ cup minced onion
1 pound ground beef
1 teaspoon minced garlic
¼ cup ketchup, or
   2 tablespoons
   tomato paste
2 tablespoons Taco
   Seasoning (page 216)
½ cup instant rice,
   white or brown
½ cup gluten-free chicken
   broth, or water
4 red bell peppers, cored
   and halved lengthwise
1 cup shredded Mexican
   cheese blend, divided

Taco night made the rounds in our family every week until we stopped eating wheat. Soft corn tortillas didn't keep all the ingredients tucked neatly inside, and the gluten-free varieties were pricey when each person wanted several tacos. This recipe brings back all the familiar flavors and is naturally gluten-free.

1. Preheat the oven to 425°F.

2. In a large skillet or sauté pan over medium-high heat, heat the olive oil.

3. Add the onion and cook for about 2 minutes, stirring, until slightly softened. Push the onion to the sides of the pan.

4. Add the ground beef to the pan and break it up with a wooden spoon. Cook for about 5 minutes until gently browned.

5. Add the garlic and cook for 30 seconds.

144   The Gluten-Free Cookbook for Families

6. Stir in the ketchup, taco seasoning, rice, and chicken broth. Bring to a simmer.

7. Evenly divide the meat mixture among the pepper halves. Top each with 2 tablespoons of cheese. Place the peppers in an 8-by-10-inch baking dish and bake for 15 to 18 minutes, or until the peppers are softened and the cheese is browned and bubbling.

SERVING TIP Serve with all the classic fixings: shredded lettuce, sliced avocado, sour cream, and corn chips.

SUBSTITUTION TIP To make this dairy-free and allergen-free, omit the shredded cheese.

PER SERVING Calories 455; Total Carbohydrates 22g; Sugar 9g; Total Fat 21g; Saturated Fat 9g; Sodium 424mg; Protein 44g; Fiber 3g

SHEPHERD'S PIE

SERVES 4 TO 6 ° PREP TIME: 5 MINUTES ° COOK TIME: 25 MINUTES

2 tablespoons canola oil

2 carrots, diced

1 yellow onion, diced

1 celery stalk, minced

2 garlic cloves, minced

1½ pounds ground beef

1 cup frozen peas

1 tablespoon tomato paste

1 teaspoon minced
fresh thyme

1 teaspoon minced
fresh rosemary

2 cups water

3 tablespoons butter

½ teaspoon sea salt

2 cups instant mashed
potato flakes

1 cup milk

This meat and potato casserole is naturally gluten-free—or so I thought. Wheat flour is sometimes used as a thickener for the meat layer in the traditional preparation. Fortunately, you don't need flour if you don't add liquid to the meat. So here is my naturally grain-free and gluten-free version.

1. Preheat the oven to 425°F.

2. In a large skillet or sauté pan over medium-high heat, heat the canola oil.

3. Add the carrots, onion, celery, and garlic and cook for 2 to 3 minutes until just beginning to soften. Push the vegetables to the sides of the pan.

4. Add the ground beef and break it up with a wooden spoon. Cook for 2 to 3 minutes. It will not be cooked through yet.

5. Stir in the peas, tomato paste, thyme, and rosemary. Bring to a simmer and cook for 1 minute. Transfer the mixture to an 8-by-10-inch baking dish.

6. While the meat and vegetables are cooking, prepare the mashed potatoes. In a medium saucepan, bring the water, butter, and salt to a simmer. Stir in the potato flakes and milk until smooth. Spread the potatoes over the meat and vegetable mixture.

7. Bake for 18 minutes, or until the potatoes are gently browned.

INGREDIENT TIP Shepherd's pie is often made with ground lamb, as its name suggests. My kids and I prefer the familiar flavor of ground beef instead.

SUBSTITUTION TIP To make this dish dairy-free and allergen-free, use nondairy butter and unsweetened nondairy milk.

PER SERVING Calories 632; Total Carbohydrates 36g; Sugar 9g; Total Fat 28g; Saturated Fat 11g; Sodium 520mg; Protein 59g; Fiber 6g

MEAT LOVER'S
Meatballs

SERVES 4 ∘ PREP TIME: 5 MINUTES ∘ COOK TIME: 25 TO 28 MINUTES

1 slice gluten-free bread,
  torn into pieces
½ cup milk
1 cup minced yellow onion
1 tablespoon
  minced garlic
1 egg, whisked
½ cup shredded
  Parmesan cheese
2 tablespoons minced
  fresh parsley
1 teaspoon minced
  fresh thyme
1 teaspoon minced
  fresh oregano
1 teaspoon sea salt
½ teaspoon freshly
  ground black pepper
¾ pound ground beef
¾ pound ground pork
2 tablespoons extra-virgin
  olive oil
3 cups gluten-free
  marinara sauce

Serve these meatballs as an entrée on their own, place them atop gluten-free pasta, or tuck them into gluten-free rolls for a meatball sandwich. I like to make the meatballs very large—about the size of my fist. However, they cook more quickly and are better for sandwiches if you make them smaller.

1. Preheat the oven to 425°F.

2. In a small bowl, combine the bread and milk. Soak for 1 minute, remove the bread, and squeeze out most of the excess moisture. Place it in a large bowl.

3. Add the onion, garlic, egg, Parmesan cheese, parsley, thyme, oregano, salt, and pepper. Stir to mix.

4. Add the beef and pork to the bowl and with your hands, mix thoroughly. Shape the mixture into 8 to 12 large balls.

5. Heat a cast-iron skillet or another ovenproof skillet over medium-high heat. Add the olive oil to the pan.

6. Add the meatballs and gently fry for about 10 minutes, browning them on all sides.

7. Pour in the marinara sauce and transfer the pan to the oven. Bake for 15 to 18 minutes until the sauce is bubbling and the meatballs are cooked through and tender.

SUBSTITUTION TIP Dried herbs work just as well in this recipe. Use half as much as you would for fresh herbs.

SERVING TIP Try serving these with naturally gluten-free "pasta": spiralized zucchini or baked spaghetti squash. Slice the spaghetti squash crosswise into 1-inch pieces, scrape out the seeds and membranes, place on a parchment-lined baking sheet, and roast for about 30 minutes.

PER SERVING Calories 603; Total Carbohydrates 33g; Sugar 19g; Total Fat 25g; Saturated Fat 8g; Sodium 1521mg; Protein 59g; Fiber 6g

BAKED LAMB
Meatballs

DAIRY-FREE
NUT-FREE

1 plum tomato,
 finely diced
½ cup minced red onion
1 tablespoon
 minced garlic
1 egg, whisked
2 tablespoons minced
 fresh parsley
1 tablespoon minced
 fresh oregano
1 teaspoon sea salt
½ teaspoon freshly
 ground black pepper
1 ½ pounds ground lamb

In this version, the meatballs are baked instead of panfried. This technique can be used with the Meat Lover's Meatballs (page 148) as well. It also swaps the bread crumbs for finely diced tomato to keep the meatballs moist. Save a few of the leftovers to serve with the Greek Salad (page 60).

1. Preheat the oven to 400°F.

2. In a large bowl, mix the tomato, onion, garlic, egg, parsley, oregano, salt, and pepper.

3. Add the lamb and, with your hands, mix thoroughly. Shape the mixture into 24 balls, and place them on a rimmed baking sheet

4. Bake for 20 minutes, or until gently browned and cooked through.

SERVING TIP Use butter lettuce leaves to make a naturally gluten-free wrap and top these meatballs with a few teaspoons of hummus, fresh grape tomatoes, and toasted pine nuts.

VARIATION TIP Serve these meatballs with the Greek Salad (page 60) and drizzle with a simple tzatziki sauce: Whisk together ½ minced cucumber, 1 cup plain Greek yogurt, zest and juice of 1 lemon, 1 teaspoon minced garlic, and 1 teaspoon minced fresh dill. Season with salt.

PER SERVING Calories 349; Total Carbohydrates 4g; Sugar 1g; Total Fat 14g; Saturated Fat 5g; Sodium 616mg; Protein 50g; Fiber 1g

NEW YORK STEAK
with Romesco Sauce

SERVES 4 ° PREP TIME: 5 MINUTES ° COOK TIME: 15 TO 18 MINUTES

DAIRY-FREE
SPLURGE-WORTHY

¼ cup extra-virgin olive
  oil, divided
4 (8-ounce) New York
  strip steaks
Sea salt
Freshly ground
  black pepper
1 slice gluten-free bread,
  crusts removed, torn
  into pieces
1 teaspoon minced garlic
Pinch red pepper flakes
2 tablespoons roughly
  chopped hazelnuts
½ cup canned diced
  fire-roasted tomatoes
2 roasted red bell peppers,
  roughly chopped
1 teaspoon ancho
  chile powder
1 tablespoon red
  wine vinegar

After cooking with tougher cuts of meat for a long time, I was pleasantly reminded how amazing New York strip steak is. The meat is cut from the short loin and is nearly as tender as the tenderloin and rib eye, but somewhat less expensive.

1. Preheat the oven to 350°F.

2. Heat a cast-iron skillet or another ovenproof skillet over medium-high heat until hot, about 2 minutes. Add 1 tablespoon of the olive oil and heat until hot but not smoking.

3. Pat the steaks dry with a paper towel and generously season both sides with salt and pepper.

4. Place the steaks into the skillet and sear for 4 minutes on each side. Transfer the skillet to the oven and finish cooking for another 3 to 5 minutes for medium-rare. (Thinner steaks will cook more quickly.)

5. Transfer the steaks to a cutting board to rest for 5 minutes while you make the romesco sauce.

152   The Gluten-Free Cookbook for Families

6. Return the skillet to medium heat and add the remaining
   3 tablespoons olive oil.

7. Add the bread, garlic, red chili flakes, and hazelnuts. Cook for 2 to
   3 minutes until golden.

8. Stir in the tomatoes, bell peppers, and ancho chile powder. Cook
   for 2 minutes. Transfer the mixture to a blender. Add the vinegar
   and purée until mostly smooth. Season with salt and pepper.

9. Spread a few tablespoons of romesco sauce onto each serving
   plate and top each with a steak.

SERVING TIP If serving this to young children, reduce the number of
steaks to 3 and split one for the kids.

COOKING TIP Be very careful when transferring the cast-iron skillet
back to the stove top. I like to set an oven mitt over the handle to remind
myself that it's hot.

PER SERVING Calories 604; Total Carbohydrates 6g; Sugar 3g; Total Fat 26g;
Saturated Fat 6g; Sodium 180mg; Protein 83mg; Fiber 2g

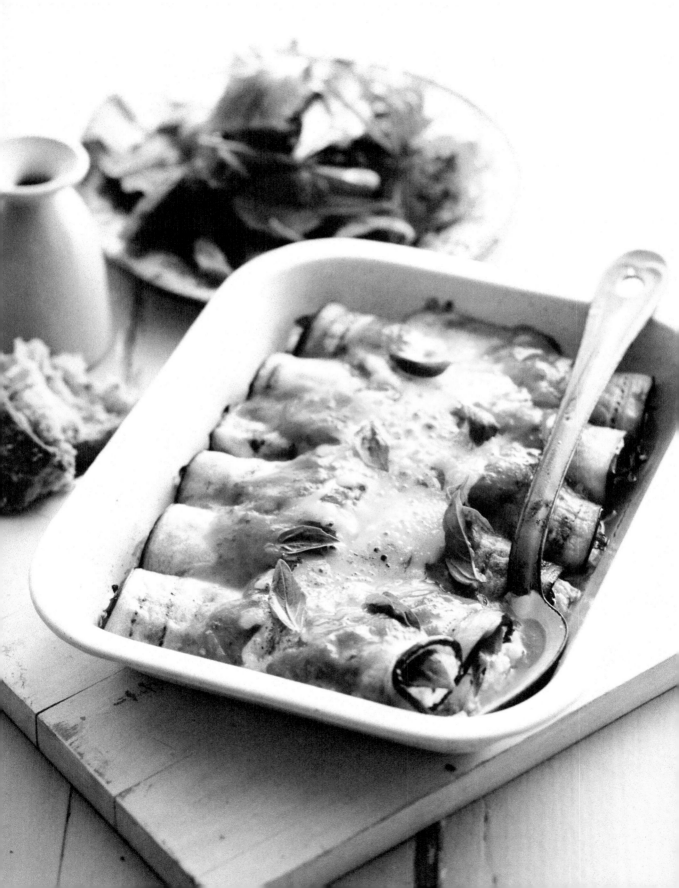

CHAPTER *Seven*

VEGETARIAN AND VEGAN

MAC 'N' CHEESE

EGG-FREE
NUT-FREE
VEGETARIAN

1 tablespoon butter

16 ounces gluten-free elbow macaroni

2 cups Cheese Sauce (White Sauce, Variation Tip with cheese, page 214)

½ cup crumbled cooked bacon (optional)

2 scallions, green parts only, thinly sliced (optional)

¼ cup minced canned jalapeño peppers (optional)

1 cup shredded Cheddar cheese

My kids love macaroni and cheese, but that goes without saying—doesn't every kid? While there are some packaged versions available with gluten-free noodles, the cheese sauce is bland and clumpy. This version is fit for kids and adults alike.

1. Preheat the broiler to high.

2. Position the oven rack about 6 inches from the element to accommodate a casserole dish.

3. Coat a 2-quart casserole dish with butter.

4. Bring a large pot of salted water to a boil over high heat. Cook the macaroni according to the package instructions. Drain and return to the pot.

5. Pour the cheese sauce over the noodles and stir to mix.

6. Fold in the bacon, scallions (if using), and jalapeños (if using).

7. Transfer the macaroni to the prepared casserole dish and top with the Cheddar cheese. Broil for 1 to 2 minutes, or until the cheese is browned and bubbling.

COOKING TIP Vary the cheeses in the sauce based on your preference.

PER SERVING Calories 811; Total Carbohydrates 97g; Sugar 9g; Total Fat 31g; Saturated Fat 19g; Sodium 585mg; Protein 36g; Fiber 4g

CORN FRITTERS

MAKES 14 TO 16 FRITTERS ∘ PREP TIME: 10 MINUTES ∘ COOK TIME: 14 MINUTES

ALLERGEN-FREE
NUT-FREE
VEGAN

½ cup garbanzo bean (chickpea) flour
2 teaspoons aluminum-free, double-acting baking powder
1 teaspoon ground cumin
1 teaspoon ground coriander
Pinch cayenne pepper
½ teaspoon sea salt
1 cup corn, either fresh kernels, or frozen and thawed
1 scallion, white and green parts, thinly sliced on the bias
½ cup nondairy milk
¼ cup extra-virgin olive oil

These savory corn fritters can be taken in many different directions. Use them as a naturally gluten-free addition to an appetizer platter. Serve them on a bed of mixed greens with lime juice and sour cream. Or, my favorite, dip them into a tangy Aioli (page 223) whipped with gluten-free adobo sauce.

1. In a large bowl, add the garbanzo bean flour, baking powder, cumin, coriander, cayenne pepper, and salt, and whisk to combine.

2. Stir in the corn and scallion.

3. Pour in the milk, whisking until no lumps remain.

4. In a large skillet or sauté pan over medium-high, heat the oil olive for 1 to 2 minutes until hot.

5. Scoop about ¼ cup of the fritter batter into the hot oil to make one fritter. Repeat with the remaining batter. You will need to do this in two batches to avoid crowding the pan. Cook for 3 minutes on each side. Transfer the cooked fritters to a cooling rack.

INGREDIENT TIP Fresh corn kernels provide a more appealing texture than frozen corn in this dish because they have a sweet pop when you bite into them.

PER SERVING Calories 72g; Total Carbohydrates 7g; Sugar 2g; Total Fat 4g; Saturated Fat 1g; Sodium 73mg; Protein 2g; Fiber 2g

TORTILLA ESPAÑOLA

SERVES 4 ∘ PREP TIME: 5 MINUTES ∘ COOK TIME: 25 MINUTES

DAIRY-FREE
NUT-FREE
ONE POT
VEGETARIAN

2 tablespoons extra-virgin
  olive oil
1 yellow onion, halved
  and thinly sliced
2 small potatoes, peeled
  and thinly cut into rounds
Sea salt
8 eggs, whisked
Freshly ground
  black pepper

Rich visited Spain on a photography assignment last year and ate this classic Spanish tapa nearly every day. When he returned, he encouraged me to add it to our menu. I like to serve it with a drizzle of Aioli (page 223) and a few side dishes that require minimal preparation, such as marinated olives, a simple kale salad, and Prosciutto-Wrapped Dates (page 87).

1. Preheat the oven to 375°F.

2. In a large skillet or sauté pan over medium heat, heat the olive oil.

3. Add the onion and potatoes. Season with a pinch salt and cook for 15 minutes, stirring often, until the potatoes are just tender.

4. Season the eggs with salt and pepper and pour them into the pan. Cook for 5 minutes, undisturbed. Transfer the pan to the oven to finish cooking for 5 minutes more, or until the eggs are set.

5. Cut into 4 wedges and serve.

INGREDIENT TIP I usually make this recipe with whatever potatoes I have on hand, usually Russets. Yukon Gold is an even better option because it has a creamier texture.

PER SERVING Calories 270; Total Carbohydrates 20g; Sugar 3g; Total Fat 16g; Saturated Fat 4g; Sodium 189mg; Protein 13g; Fiber 3g

VEGAN CHILI

SERVES 4 ° PREP TIME: 10 MINUTES ° COOK TIME: 20 MINUTES

ALLERGEN-FREE
NUT-FREE
ONE POT
SLOW COOKER OPTION
VEGAN

2 tablespoons canola oil
2 carrots, diced
2 celery stalks,
  finely diced
1 yellow onion, diced
2 cups sliced button
  mushrooms
4 garlic cloves, minced
2 (15-ounce) cans pinto
  or cannellini beans,
  drained and rinsed
2 (15-ounce) cans diced
  fire-roasted tomatoes
¼ cup Taco Seasoning
  (page 216)
Sea salt
Freshly ground
  black pepper
2 avocados, thinly sliced

It might seem strange to use taco seasoning in chili, but many of the spices are identical, and sometimes it's just nice to have everything premixed and ready to go. See the Ingredient Tip for how much of each spice to use in this recipe.

1. In a large pot over medium heat, heat the canola oil.

2. Add the carrots, celery, and onion and cook for about 5 minutes until the vegetables begin to soften.

3. Push the vegetables to the sides of the pan and add the mushrooms. Cook for 3 minutes until they release some of their liquid.

4. Stir in the garlic and cook for 30 seconds.

5. Add the beans, tomatoes, and taco seasoning. Season with salt and pepper and simmer, uncovered, for 20 minutes.

6. Serve with the avocado slices.

INGREDIENT TIP If you don't have a batch of Taco Seasoning already mixed, use 1 tablespoon ground cumin, 1 tablespoon smoked paprika, 1 tablespoon ancho chile powder, ½ teaspoon onion powder, ½ teaspoon garlic powder, ¼ teaspoon ground oregano, and a pinch cayenne pepper. Store in a sealed jar in a dark place.

SLOW COOKER OPTION To make this in a slow cooker, place all the ingredients into the cooker *except* the avocado slices. Cover and for 6 to 8 hours cook on low. Serve with the avocado slices.

PER SERVING Calories 696; Total Carbohydrates 89g; Sugar 12g; Total Fat 28g; Saturated Fat 5g; Sodium 190mg; Protein 31g; Fiber 38g

SAUTÉED LEEK
and Mushroom Flatbreads

SERVES 2 • PREP TIME: 5 MINUTES PLUS 10 MINUTES INACTIVE TIME
COOK TIME: 15 MINUTES

MAKE DAIRY-FREE
MAKE VEGAN

FOR THE CRUST
1 ½ teaspoons sugar
⅓ cup hot water (<110°F)
1 package (2 ¼ teaspoons)
  active dry yeast
1 cup finely ground
  blanched almond flour
¾ cup tapioca flour
  (starch)
¾ teaspoon sea salt
1 egg white
1 ½ teaspoons red
  wine vinegar
¼ cup potato starch
1 to 2 tablespoons extra-
  virgin olive oil

FOR THE TOPPINGS
1 tablespoon extra-virgin
  olive oil
1 yellow onion, very
  thinly sliced
Sea salt
2 tablespoons butter
2 cups thinly sliced
  mushrooms
1 leek, white and green
  parts, thinly cut into
  half circles
¼ cup balsamic vinegar
Freshly ground
  black pepper

A similar recipe appears in Chef Candice Kumai's cookbook, *Cook Yourself Sexy*. Garnish with lots of grated Parmesan cheese and fresh basil leaves before serving.

1. Preheat the oven to 425°F.

2. Place a pizza stone or pizza pan into the oven to heat.

TO MAKE THE CRUST

1. In a small bowl, stir together the sugar and hot water to dissolve the sugar. Add the yeast and whisk with a fork to disburse the yeast granules. Set aside.

2. In a medium bowl, mix the almond flour, tapioca flour, and salt. Make a well in the center of the ingredients. Add the egg white and vinegar.

3. The yeast should be foamy by now. Pour it into the mixing bowl and stir to combine. The dough will be quite wet.

4. Add the potato starch and stir to mix thoroughly.

5. Turn out the dough onto a large sheet of parchment paper and spread it into two rectangles with a spatula. It will be much wetter than traditional pizza dough.

6. Pour the extra-virgin olive oil onto the flatbread dough and your clean hands. Press the dough into two 8-inch rectangles. Gently press down with your fingertips to create small divots in the crust. Let it rest for 15 minutes.

7. Slide the flatbreads and parchment paper onto the preheated pizza stone. Bake for 10 minutes until puffy and golden brown.

TO MAKE THE TOPPINGS

1. While the crust is resting and baking, in a large skillet or sauté pan over medium heat, heat the extra-virgin olive oil.

2. Add the onion and a pinch salt. Cook, stirring, for 10 to 12 minutes until gently browned. Push the onions to the sides of the pan.

3. In the center of the pan, melt the butter.

4. Add the mushrooms and sauté until browned on both sides, about 8 minutes total. You may want to do this in two batches so as not to crowd the pan.

5. Stir the leek into the pan to combine the ingredients.

6. Pour in the vinegar and simmer for 3 to 5 minutes until the vinegar is reduced. Season with pepper.

7. Remove the pizza from the oven and top with the vegetable mixture.

SUBSTITUTION TIP To make this flatbread vegan and dairy-free, use evaporated cane juice in place of the white sugar and a vegan egg replacer in the dough. Omit the butter.

PER SERVING Calories 737; Total Carbohydrates 63g; Sugar 12g; Total Fat 50g; Saturated Fat 11g; Sodium 937mg; Protein 17g; Fiber 10g

LOADED VEGETARIAN PIZZA

SERVES 2 ∘ PREP TIME: 5 MINUTES PLUS 10 MINUTES INACTIVE TIME
COOK TIME: 15 MINUTES

NUT-FREE
VEGETARIAN
MAKE DAIRY-FREE

FOR THE CRUST
1 ½ teaspoons sugar
⅓ cup hot water (<110°F)
1 package (2 ¼ teaspoons)
  active dry yeast
1 cup finely ground
  blanched almond flour
¾ cup tapioca flour (starch)
¾ teaspoon sea salt
1 egg white
1 ½ teaspoons red
  wine vinegar
¼ cup potato starch
1 to 2 tablespoons
  extra-virgin olive oil

FOR THE TOPPINGS
1 tablespoon butter
1 cup thinly sliced
  mushrooms
1 cup marinara sauce
1 roasted red pepper,
  thinly sliced
1 large heirloom tomato,
  thinly sliced
1 (4-ounce) ball fresh
  mozzarella, thinly
  sliced (optional)
½ cup fresh basil leaves

I didn't think it was possible to make a pizza crust—let alone a gluten-free pizza crust—in just 30 minutes. Then this happened: the best gluten-free pizza I have ever had. Seriously. Stop whatever you're doing and go make this pizza. Top it with whatever you like—even just olive oil, a few slices of fresh mozzarella, and tomatoes is heaven. This recipe yields one 12-inch pizza. For my family, we make two and are satisfied.

1. Preheat the oven to 425°F.

2. Place a pizza stone or pizza pan into the oven to heat.

TO MAKE THE CRUST

1. In a small bowl, stir together the sugar and hot water to dissolve the sugar. Add the yeast and whisk with a fork to disburse the yeast granules. Set aside.

2. In a medium bowl, mix the almond flour, tapioca flour, and salt. Make a well in the center of the ingredients and add the egg white and vinegar.

3. The yeast should be foamy by now. Pour it into the bowl and stir to combine. The dough will be quite wet.

4. Add the potato starch and stir to mix thoroughly.

5. Turn out the dough onto a large sheet of parchment paper and spread it into a small circle with a spatula. It will be much wetter than traditional pizza dough.

6. Pour the olive oil onto the pizza dough and your clean hands. With your hands, press the dough into a 12-inch circle. Use your palms to press the center of the dough down and gently nudge the sides of the dough to be somewhat thicker. Let rest for 10 minutes.

7. Slide the pizza dough and parchment paper onto the preheated pizza stone. Bake for 5 minutes.

TO MAKE THE TOPPINGS

1. While the pizza is resting and baking, in a large skillet or sauté pan over medium-high heat, melt the butter. Add the mushrooms and sauté until browned on both sides, about 5 minutes.

2. Remove the pizza from the oven. Cover with the marinara sauce, sautéed mushrooms, red pepper, tomato, and mozzarella cheese (if using).

3. Return to the oven to bake for 8 to 10 minutes more until the cheese is melted and gently browned.

4. Top with the fresh basil leaves and serve.

SUBSTITUTION TIP To make this recipe dairy-free, use olive oil in place of the butter and omit the cheese.

PER SERVING Calories 859; Total Carbohydrates 74g; Sugar 21g; Total Fat 51g; Saturated Fat 14g; Sodium 1626mg; Protein 34g; Fiber 13g

SPINACH AND
Black Bean Enchiladas

SERVES 4 TO 6 ° PREP TIME: 5 MINUTES ° COOK TIME: 25 MINUTES

EGG-FREE
NUT-FREE
VEGETARIAN

1 tablespoon extra-virgin
  olive oil
1 yellow onion, minced
2 garlic cloves, minced
8 cups shredded fresh
  spinach
1 (15-ounce) can
  black beans, rinsed
  and drained
1 (8-ounce) package
  cream cheese
1 tablespoon
  ground cumin
1 teaspoon smoked
  paprika
2 cups shredded Mexican
  cheese blend, divided
2 cups Enchilada
  Sauce (page 217), or
  1 (15-ounce) can gluten-
  free enchilada sauce
12 gluten-free
  corn tortillas
Sour cream, for
  serving (optional)
¼ cup roughly chopped
  fresh cilantro (optional)

This is one of Rich's favorite dinners and it is equally popular with everyone I share it with. If you're not used to cooking with cumin, be prepared—it has a pungent aroma. But the taste is traditional and perfectly offset by the velvety cream cheese filling.

1. Preheat the oven to 400°F.

2. In a large skillet or sauté pan over medium heat, heat the olive oil.

3. Add the onion and garlic and cook, stirring frequently, for 2 to 3 minutes until just beginning to soften.

4. Stir in the spinach and black beans. Cook for 1 to 2 minutes until the spinach is wilted and begins to release its liquid.

5. Add the cream cheese, cumin, and paprika. Stir until the cream cheese is softened and integrated with the spinach and black beans. Remove the pan from the heat. Stir in 1½ cups of the shredded cheese.

6. Cover the bottom of an 8-by-10-inch baking dish with ½ cup of the enchilada sauce.

7. Lay out the tortillas on the work surface and evenly divide the filling among them. Roll each into a cylinder. Arrange them seam-side down in the baking dish.

8. Pour the remaining enchilada sauce over the tortillas and sprinkle with the remaining ½ cup shredded cheese. Bake for 15 to 20 minutes, or until the cheese is bubbling and the filling is hot.

9. Serve with sour cream (if using) and fresh cilantro (if using).

COOKING TIP You can make this dish ahead of time and refrigerate it until ready to bake. Increase the baking time by about 10 minutes if baking straight from the refrigerator.

PER SERVING Calories 768; Total Carbohydrates 83g; Sugar 10g; Total Fat 35g; Saturated Fat 17g; Sodium 1220mg; Protein 38g; Fiber 17g

VEGETARIAN LASAGNA

SERVES 4 ∘ PREP TIME: 5 MINUTES ∘ COOK TIME: 25 MINUTES

NUT-FREE
SPLURGE-WORTHY
VEGETARIAN

1 (16-ounce) container
  ricotta cheese
1 egg, whisked
1 teaspoon dried oregano
2 cups shredded
  mozzarella cheese
4 cups shredded Italian
  cheese blend, divided
1 (9-ounce) package
  oven-ready gluten-free
  lasagna noodles
2½ cups gluten-free
  marinara sauce
2 cups loosely packed
  fresh basil leaves

This rich vegetarian lasagna is so delicious it even wins over avowed meat lovers. The basil is what really makes it, so don't skimp.

1. Preheat the oven to 375°F.

2. In a medium bowl, mix the ricotta, egg, oregano, mozzarella, and 1½ cups of Italian cheese blend.

3. Cover the bottom of a large glass baking dish with 1 cup marinara sauce.

4. Place a layer of noodles over the sauce, and top with 1 cup marinara. Brush to coat the noodles.

5. Cover with ½ cup of the remaining Italian cheese mixture and a handful of fresh basil.

6. Repeat, building two more layers with the noodles, sauce, cheese, and basil as described in steps 4 and 5.

7. Finish with a ½-cup layer of marinara. Top with the remaining 1 cup shredded Italian cheese and a sprinkle of fresh basil.

8. Bake for 25 minutes, uncovered, or until the cheese is browned and bubbling.

INGREDIENT TIP Choose "oven-ready" lasagna noodles that do not need to be preboiled. If possible, use a baking dish that easily accommodates the brand of noodles you have without needing to break them to fit. Some noodles have the traditional long rectangle shape with fluted sides, for which an 8-by-10-inch pan works well.

PER SERVING Calories 875; Total Carbohydrates 78g; Sugar 23g; Total Fat 29g; Saturated Fat 14g; Sodium 2533mg; Protein 73g; Fiber 7g

ROASTED RED PEPPER
and Hummus Sandwiches

SERVES 4 ° PREP TIME: 5 MINUTES

NUT-FREE
VEGETARIAN

1 cup prepared hummus
4 gluten-free rolls,
 halved, or 8 slices
 gluten-free bread
2 roasted red bell
 peppers, sliced
4 thick slices
 Havarti cheese
1 cup arugula

This recipe could just as easily make a lovely lunch, but I think it makes an even more delectable picnic dinner. Store all the ingredients separately and assemble the sandwiches when you're ready to eat. This also gives those who want a dairy-free option the chance to make their own sandwich.

1. Spread ¼ cup of the hummus onto the bottom half of each roll.

2. Top with the bell pepper, Havarti, and arugula. Serve immediately.

COOKING TIP For even more roasted red pepper flavor, in a blender, combine the hummus with 1 roasted red pepper, 1 garlic clove, and 1 teaspoon freshly squeezed lemon juice and purée until smooth.

PER SERVING Calories 299; Total Carbohydrates 35g; Sugar 6g; Total Fat 13g; Saturated Fat 4g; Sodium 533mg; Protein 13g; Fiber 6g

BARBECUED TOFU BURGERS

SERVES 4 ° PREP TIME: 5 MINUTES ° COOK TIME: 12 MINUTES

NUT-FREE
VEGETARIAN

1 tablespoon canola oil
1 (16-ounce) tofu block,
    halved horizontally
    and pressed (see
    Ingredient Tip)
2 cups Barbecue Sauce
    (page 215), or store-
    bought gluten-free
    barbecue sauce
4 gluten-free
    hamburger buns
4 slices pepper Jack
    cheese (optional)
1 red onion, thinly sliced
    into rings
1 cup shredded
    romaine lettuce

Everything is right about this vegetarian burger.
I prefer the Trader Joe's brand of gluten-free
hamburger buns because they don't fall apart.

1. In a large skillet or sauté pan over medium-high heat,
   heat the canola oil until hot.

2. Pat the tofu slices dry with paper towels and place them
   into the hot pan. Cook for 4 minutes on each side to
   develop a golden-brown crust.

3. Transfer the cooked tofu slices to a cutting board and cut
   each into about 6 slices. Return to the pan and reduce
   the heat to low.

4. Add the barbecue sauce and cook the tofu and sauce for
   about 2 minutes until the sauce is heated through. Set aside.

5. Preheat the broiler.

6. Place the hamburger buns under the broiler for about
   2 minutes to toast gently—watch them carefully.

7. Place several slices of tofu with sauce on the bottom half
   of each bun and top with a slice of pepper Jack cheese
   (if using). Top each with a few onion rings and a handful
   of lettuce.

INGREDIENT TIP To press the tofu, slice it in half horizontally.
Place it between two rimmed pans or pie plates. Set a weight on
the top plate to press out excess moisture. Press 5 minutes to
30 minutes.

PER SERVING Calories 479; Total Carbohydrates 72g; Sugar 37g;
Total Fat 13g; Saturated Fat 3g; Sodium 1792mg; Protein 21g; Fiber 3g

VEGAN SLOPPY JOES

SERVES 4 ° PREP TIME: 5 MINUTES ° COOK TIME: 15 MINUTES

ALLERGEN-FREE
NUT-FREE
ONE POT
SLOW COOKER OPTION
VEGAN

2 tablespoons canola oil
1 yellow onion, minced
2 garlic cloves, smashed
Sea salt
2 (8-ounce) packages
  tempeh, crumbled
1 roasted red bell
  pepper, diced
1 (15-ounce) can
  tomato sauce
2 tablespoons
  brown sugar
1 tablespoon red
  wine vinegar
1 tablespoon vegan
  Worcestershire sauce
1 teaspoon
  smoked paprika
Freshly ground
  black pepper
4 gluten-free rolls, halved

It's not the meat that keeps me coming back to this childhood favorite—it's the sauce! This version uses crumbled tempeh to mimic the texture of ground beef. This dish is especially kid friendly—just be sure have an extra stack of napkins nearby.

1. In a large skillet or sauté pan over medium heat, heat the canola oil.

2. Add the onion, garlic, and a pinch salt. Cook for about 5 minutes, stirring often, until soft. Push the onion and garlic to the sides of the pan.

3. Add the tempeh to the pan and cook for 5 minutes until browned.

4. Stir in the roasted red pepper, tomato sauce, brown sugar, vinegar, Worcestershire sauce, and paprika. Season with salt and pepper. Cook for 5 minutes to allow the flavors to come together.

5. Top each roll with a generous scoop of the tempeh mixture and serve.

INGREDIENT TIP Most gluten-free breads are leavened with eggs. If you are vegan or cannot eat eggs, look for vegan, gluten-free rolls. The Schar brand is one option. It is shelf stable and stored in plastic packaging.

SLOW COOKER OPTION To make this recipe in a slow cooker, place all the ingredients *except* the buns into a slow cooker. Cover and cook for 6 hours on low.

PER SERVING Calories 472; Total Carbohydrates 48g; Sugar 14g; Total Fat 22g; Saturated Fat 4g; Sodium 877mg; Protein; Fiber 4g

FRIED GREEN TOMATO
Sandwiches

SERVES 4 ° PREP TIME: 5 MINUTES ° COOK TIME: 16 MINUTES

DAIRY-FREE
NUT-FREE
VEGETARIAN
MAKE VEGAN

FOR THE FRIED GREEN TOMATOES
2 tablespoons canola oil
1 egg white
Sea salt
Freshly ground
  black pepper
1 cup cornmeal
2 large green tomatoes, cut
  into ¼-inch-thick slices

FOR THE COLESLAW
¼ cup mayonnaise
1 tablespoon freshly
  squeezed lemon juice
1 teaspoon ground cumin
4 cups shredded cabbage
1 Granny Smith apple,
  unpeeled and julienned
½ red onion, thinly sliced

FOR ASSEMBLY
8 slices gluten-free
  bread, toasted
1 cup Barbecue Sauce
  (page 215), or store-
  bought gluten-free
  barbecue sauce

The flavors in this vegetarian sandwich are transformative—the crunchy, crusty tomatoes with creamy coleslaw and tangy barbecue sauce take me to another place. What are you waiting for?

TO MAKE THE FRIED GREEN TOMATOES

1. In a large skillet or sauté pan over medium-high heat, heat the canola oil.

2. In a small, shallow bowl, season the egg white with salt and pepper and whisk to combine.

3. Place the cornmeal in another small, shallow bowl.

4. Dip each tomato slice into the egg white and then dredge it in the cornmeal. Place it in the hot skillet and fry for 3 to 4 minutes on each side. You will need to do this in batches.

TO MAKE THE COLESLAW

1. In a large bowl, whisk the mayonnaise, lemon juice, and cumin.

2. Add the cabbage, apple, and onion and gently toss to combine.

TO ASSEMBLE THE SANDWICHES

1. Place the slices of fried green tomato on 4 slices of bread.

2. Top each with a spoonful of barbecue sauce and then finish with the coleslaw. Top each with another slice of bread. Serve immediately.

SUBSTITUTION TIP To make this dish vegan, use 1 flax egg (1 tablespoon water mixed with 1 tablespoon ground flax meal) in place of the egg white, use a vegan mayonnaise, and vegan gluten-free bread or rolls.

PER SERVING Calories 295; Total Carbohydrates 41g; Sugar 11g; Total Fat 13g; Saturated Fat 2g; Sodium 200mg; Protein 5g; Fiber 6g

EGGPLANT INVOLTINI

SERVES 4 ◦ PREP TIME: 5 MINUTES ◦ COOK TIME: 25 MINUTES

EGG-FREE
MAKE NUT-FREE
MAKE VEGAN

2 medium eggplant,
  stem ends removed and
  sliced lengthwise into
  ¼-inch-thick slices
¼ cup extra-virgin olive oil
Sea salt
8 ounces crumbled
  feta cheese
2 tablespoons roughly
  chopped raisins
2 tablespoons roughly
  chopped toasted pine
  nuts (optional)
2 garlic cloves, minced
2 tablespoons minced
  fresh parsley
1 tablespoon minced
  fresh mint
Zest of 1 lemon
Freshly ground
  black pepper
1½ cups tomato
  purée, divided
1 cup shredded
  mozzarella cheese
¼ cup fresh basil leaves

This light dinner is loosely related to lasagna, but much lower in carbohydrates. I like to serve it with a simple side salad or Grain-Free Breadsticks (page 88).

1. Preheat the oven to 375°F.

2. Heat a large skillet or griddle over medium heat.

3. Brush the eggplant slices with olive oil and season with salt. Place the slices in the skillet and cook for about 5 minutes until slightly softened. Set aside to cool slightly.

4. While the eggplant cooks, in a medium bowl, mix the feta cheese, raisins, pine nuts, garlic, parsley, mint, and lemon zest. Season with salt and pepper.

5. Cover the bottom of a 2-quart baking dish with ½ cup of the tomato purée.

6. When the eggplant slices are cool enough to handle, spoon about 2 tablespoons of the feta mixture onto each and roll into a tight cylinder. Place them seam-side down into the baking dish.

7. Pour the remaining 1 cup tomato purée over the eggplant rolls. Sprinkle the mozzarella cheese over the top and bake for 20 minutes, or until heated through and soft.

8. Garnish with the basil and serve.

SUBSTITUTION TIP For a nut-free dish, omit the pine nuts. To make this dish vegan, skip the mozzarella topping and use an almond-milk ricotta cheese instead of the feta. To make this, in a blender, process 1 cup blanched almonds, ½ cup water, 1 teaspoon white wine vinegar or freshly squeezed lemon juice, and ¼ teaspoon sea salt until mostly smooth. Transfer the mixture to a nut-milk bag or layered cheesecloth and press out the excess moisture.

PER SERVING Calories 446; Total Carbohydrates 29g; Sugar 17g; Total Fat 30g; Saturated Fat 13g; Sodium 1351mg; Protein 20g; Fiber 11g

PLANTAIN AND BLACK BEAN BOWLS
with Collard Greens

SERVES 4 ° PREP TIME: 5 MINUTES ° COOK TIME: 24 MINUTES

ALLERGEN-FREE
NUT-FREE
VEGAN

1 (15-ounce) can
black beans, drained
and rinsed

1 teaspoon smoked
paprika

2 teaspoons minced
garlic, divided

2 tablespoons coconut oil,
or canola oil

2 barely ripe plantains,
peeled and cut into
¼-inch-thick slices

1 bunch collard greens,
thick ribs removed,
cut into thin ribbons

1 lime, halved

Although they look remarkably like bananas, plantains have a nutty flavor and are less sweet, even when fully ripe. Use barely ripe plantains for this recipe. They should be yellow but not yet spotted with black. The recipe is naturally vegan, but if you eat eggs, it is delicious topped with a drizzle of Aioli (page 223).

1. In a small saucepan over medium heat, mix the black beans, paprika, and 1 teaspoon of the garlic. Bring to a gentle simmer and cook for 5 minutes.

2. While the beans cook, in a large skillet or sauté pan over medium-high heat, heat 1 tablespoon of coconut oil until hot but not smoking. Add the plantains and panfry for 3 to 4 minutes on each side. You will likely need to do this in two batches so as not to crowd the pan. Transfer the plantains to 4 individual plates.

3. Evenly divide the black beans among the dishes.

4. In the same skillet, heat the remaining 1 tablespoon coconut oil.

5. Add the collard greens and cook for 1 to 2 minutes until bright green but still crisp.

6. Add the remaining 1 teaspoon garlic and sauté for 30 seconds more. Evenly divide the collards among the serving dishes.

7. Sprinkle each bowl with a squeeze of lime juice.

INGREDIENT TIP I prefer to use refined coconut oil (which has an indistinguishable flavor) in panfrying. However, I understand not everyone stocks this in their kitchens. Use canola oil or another neutral oil in its place.

PER SERVING Calories 234; Total Carbohydrates 41g; Sugar 14g; Total Fat 8g; Saturated Fat 1g; Sodium 196mg; Protein 5g; Fiber 6g

SWEET POTATO AND TEMPEH
Mole Bowls

SERVES 4 ○ PREP TIME: 5 MINUTES ○ COOK TIME: 25 MINUTES

VEGAN

2 large sweet potatoes,
  cut into ½-inch dice
2 tablespoons canola oil
Sea salt
½ cup sesame seeds
½ cup blanched almonds
2 gluten-free corn tortillas
¼ cup minced raisins
1 tablespoon ancho
  chile powder
¼ teaspoon ground cloves
¼ teaspoon ground
  cinnamon
¼ teaspoon red
  pepper flakes
⅛ teaspoon
  ground allspice
⅛ teaspoon ground
  coriander
2 tablespoons
  tomato paste
3 cups gluten-free
  vegetable broth, divided
3 ounces dark chocolate,
  at least 60 percent
  cacao, grated
1 (8-ounce) package
  tempeh, cut into
  2-inch pieces

I realize I am about to commit mole sacrilege here, pairing mole sauce with tempeh, and I'm sorry. Almost. Once you taste this complex, savory sauce with this neutral partner, you'll see what I mean. Tempeh is made from fermented soybeans and many people find it easier to digest than tofu.

1. Preheat the oven to 400°F.

2. Spread the sweet potatoes on a rimmed baking sheet and drizzle with the canola oil. Gently toss to coat. Season with salt and roast for 25 minutes.

3. While the sweet potatoes roast, make the mole. In a dry skillet over medium heat, toast the sesame seeds for about 2 minutes until fragrant. Transfer them to a blender.

4. To the blender, add the almonds, tortillas, raisins, ancho chile powder, cloves, cinnamon, red pepper flakes, allspice, coriander, tomato paste, and 1 cup of the vegetable broth. Purée the sauce until smooth.

5. Transfer the sauce to a medium saucepan over medium heat. Stir in the remaining 2 cups vegetable broth and bring to a simmer. Cook for 10 minutes until the mixture begins to thicken.

6. Stir in the dark chocolate and cook for 2 to 3 minutes until melted.

7. Add the tempeh pieces and cook just until heated through.

8. Evenly divide the roasted sweet potatoes among 4 serving bowls and top each with tempeh and mole sauce.

INGREDIENT TIP You can purchase mole sauce, but read the label because many kinds contain wheat flour or crackers as a thickener. Also, to ensure the dark chocolate is dairy-free, read its label, as well.

PER SERVING Calories 723; Total Carbohydrates 81g; Sugar 19g; Total Fat 36g; Saturated Fat 8g; Sodium 683mg; Protein 25g; Fiber 12g

ROASTED KABOCHA SQUASH
over Quinoa

SERVES 4 ° PREP TIME: 5 MINUTES ° COOK TIME: 25 MINUTES

ALLERGEN-FREE
NUT-FREE
VEGAN

1 kabocha squash, cubed
2 tablespoons coconut oil, melted, or canola oil
Sea salt
1 cup quinoa, rinsed and drained
2 cups vegetable broth, or water
1 cup pomegranate arils (the yield from 1 pomegranate)
¼ cup minced red onion
2 tablespoons roughly chopped fresh mint
2 tablespoons roughly chopped fresh parsley
1 tablespoon red wine vinegar
Freshly ground black pepper

When kabocha squash is roasted, the flesh becomes soft, earthy, and sweet. The skin caramelizes and provides a chewy textural contrast.

1. Preheat the oven to 425°F.

2. Spread the kabocha squash on a rimmed baking sheet and drizzle with the coconut oil. Gently toss to coat. Season with salt and roast for 25 minutes.

3. In a small saucepan over medium heat, bring the quinoa and vegetable broth to a simmer. Reduce heat to low, cover, and cook for 20 minutes, or until the quinoa has absorbed all the liquid. Fluff with a fork.

4. While the quinoa and kabocha cook, in a small bowl, combine the pomegranate arils, onion, mint, and parsley. Drizzle with the vinegar. Season with salt and pepper.

5. Evenly divide the quinoa among 4 serving bowls. Top each with kabocha squash and a generous spoonful of the pomegranate and herb mixture.

TO SAVE TIME Purchase pomegranate arils from the refrigerated section of the grocery store. Otherwise, to open a pomegranate, halve it vertically and carefully invert the skin, gently removing the seeds with your fingers.

PER SERVING Calories 344; Total Carbohydrates 59g; Sugar 10g; Total Fat 10g; Saturated Fat 1g; Sodium 75mg; Protein 9g; Fiber 8g

FETTUCCINE ALFREDO
with Peas, Edamame, and Parmesan

SERVES 4 ° PREP TIME: 5 MINUTES ° COOK TIME: 10 MINUTES

EGG-FREE
NUT-FREE
VEGETARIAN

16 ounces gluten-free
  fettuccine
2 cups White Sauce
  (page 214)
1 teaspoon minced garlic
1 cup grated Parmesan
  cheese, divided
1 cup frozen blanched
  peas, defrosted in warm
  water and drained
1 cup frozen blanched,
  shelled edamame,
  defrosted in warm water
  and drained
1 bunch fresh chives,
  sliced into 1-inch pieces
Freshly ground black
  pepper, for seasoning

Peas and edamame are good sources of protein and fiber and add beautiful color to this classic dish, which typically includes shrimp or chicken. For the best flavor, purchase a block of good-quality aged Parmesan and grate it yourself. If you happen to have roasted garlic on hand, use that in place of the fresh minced garlic.

1. Bring a large pot of salted water to a boil over high heat. Add the fettuccine and cook according to the package instructions. Drain and return to the pot.

2. Add the White Sauce, garlic, and ½ cup of Parmesan. Stir to mix.

3. Gently fold in the peas and edamame.

4. To serve, garnish with the remaining ½ cup of Parmesan and chives; season to taste with pepper.

INGREDIENT TIP If you cannot find gluten-free fettucine, use gluten-free linguine or spaghetti instead.

PER SERVING Calories 749; Total Carbohydrates 105g; Sugar 12g; Total Fat 21g; Saturated Fat 12g; Sodium 604mg; Protein 34g; Fiber 7g

POLENTA WITH ROASTED TOMATOES,
Garlic, and Greens

SERVES 4 ∘ PREP TIME: 5 MINUTES ∘ COOK TIME: 20 TO 25 MINUTES

ALLERGEN-FREE
NUT-FREE
VEGAN

16 ounces grape
  tomatoes, or cherry
  tomatoes
12 garlic cloves, peeled
¼ cup extra-virgin
  olive oil, divided
Sea salt
Freshly ground
  black pepper
3 cups vegetable broth
1 cup yellow cornmeal
6 cups fresh spinach,
  roughly chopped
1 tablespoon sherry
  vinegar, or balsamic
  vinegar

The bliss-bowl concept works especially well for vegetarian meals. Begin with a starch and top with flavorful vegetables and plant protein. The options are endless. Roasted tomatoes and garlic are especially delicious over this creamy vegan polenta.

1. Preheat the oven to 375°F.

2. Spread the tomatoes and garlic on a rimmed baking sheet. Drizzle with 2 tablespoons of the olive oil and season with salt and pepper. Roast for 20 to 25 minutes, or until the tomatoes are wilted and the garlic is soft.

3. Meanwhile, in a medium pot over medium-low heat, bring the vegetable broth, with a generous pinch salt, to a simmer.

4. While whisking constantly, pour in the cornmeal in a thin, steady stream. Reduce the heat to low and continue stirring for about 15 minutes until the mixture is thick.

5. In a separate skillet, cook the spinach with 1 tablespoon of the olive oil for about 5 minutes until it is soft. Season with salt and pepper.

6. Evenly divide the polenta among 4 serving bowls. Top each with a generous scoop of the roasted tomatoes and garlic. Serve the spinach on the side topped with a splash of vinegar. Drizzle with the remaining 1 tablespoon olive oil.

PER SERVING Calories 292; Total Carbohydrates 33g; Sugar 4g; Total Fat 15g; Saturated Fat 2g; Sodium 684mg; Protein 9g; Fiber 5g

SARDINIAN MINESTRONE

SERVES 4 TO 6 ° PREP TIME: 5 MINUTES ° COOK TIME: 20 MINUTES

EGG-FREE
NUT-FREE
ONE POT
SLOW COOKER OPTION
MAKE ALLERGEN-FREE
MAKE DAIRY-FREE
MAKE VEGAN

½ cup extra-virgin
  olive oil, divided
4 garlic cloves, smashed
2 carrots, diced
2 celery stalks, diced
1 yellow onion, diced
1 (28-ounce) can plum
  tomatoes, hand crushed
3 small yellow potatoes,
  peeled and diced
½ fennel bulb, cored
  and diced
1 (15-ounce) can
  fava beans, rinsed
  and drained
32 ounces (4 cups)
  vegetable broth
Sea salt
Freshly ground
  black pepper
8 ounces gluten-free
  shell pasta
2 tablespoons roughly
  chopped fresh parsley
¼ cup roughly chopped
  fresh basil
2 ounces shaved Pecorino
  Romano cheese
  (optional)

Sardinia is lauded for having some of the longest-lived people on Earth. That's as good a reason as any to make soup. But the taste will keep you making it again and again. This recipe uses a lot of olive oil, but that is one of the secrets to Sardinian longevity.

1. In a large pot over medium heat, heat 2 tablespoons of the olive oil.

2. Add the garlic, carrots, celery, and onion and cook for about 5 minutes until fragrant and beginning to soften.

3. Stir in the tomatoes, potatoes, fennel, fava beans, and vegetable broth. Season with salt and pepper. Bring to a simmer and cook for 5 minutes.

4. Stir in the pasta, parsley, and basil. Cook for 10 minutes more, or until the pasta is al dente.

5. Ladle the soup into serving bowls, drizzle each with about 1 tablespoon of the remaining olive oil, and top with the Pecorino Romano cheese (if using).

INGREDIENT TIP To make this an allergen-free, dairy-free, and vegan dish, omit the cheese. Pecorino Romano is a flavorful sheep's milk cheese and is loaded with healthy antioxidants. If you cannot find it, use Parmesan cheese instead. For a vegan dish, omit the cheese.

SLOW COOKER OPTION To make this in a slow cooker, add all of the ingredients *except* the cheese and 6 tablespoons of olive oil to a 4-quart slow cooker. Cover and cook for 6 to 8 hours on low.

PER SERVING Calories 770; Total Carbohydrates 102g; Sugar 13g; Total Fat 29g; Saturated Fat 4g; Sodium 2252mg; Protein 30g; Fiber 21g

HOISIN-GLAZED TOFU
and Green Beans

SERVES 4 ° PREP TIME: 15 MINUTES ° COOK TIME: 15 MINUTES

NUT-FREE
ONE POT
VEGAN

1 tablespoon canola oil

1 teaspoon toasted
sesame oil

1 (16-ounce) tofu block,
halved horizontally and
pressed (see Ingredient
Tip, page 168)

1 pound green
beans, trimmed

1 tablespoon minced
peeled fresh ginger

1 teaspoon minced garlic

Pinch red pepper flakes

¼ cup gluten-free
hoisin sauce

2 tablespoons freshly
squeezed lime juice

2 tablespoons gluten-free
soy sauce

Sea salt

Freshly ground
black pepper

6 cups steamed rice

Like so many recipes, the sauce really carries this dish. Sometimes I double the sauce because I love it so much. Definitely read the labels to ensure you use a gluten-free hoisin sauce.

1. In a large skillet or sauté pan over medium-high heat, heat the canola oil and sesame oil.

2. Pat the tofu dry with paper towels. Add it to the skillet and sear on each side for about 4 minutes to develop a nice golden crust. Transfer the cooked tofu to a cutting board to rest.

3. Return the skillet to the heat and add the green beans. Sauté for 5 minutes, or until bright green and nearly tender.

4. Add the ginger, garlic, and red pepper flakes. Cook for about 1 minute until fragrant.

5. Cut the tofu into cubes and return it to the pan.

6. In a sealable jar, combine the hoisin sauce, lime juice, and soy sauce. Seal the lid and shake vigorously to mix the ingredients. Pour the sauce into the pan and simmer for 1 minute.

7. Serve with steamed rice.

PER SERVING Calories 707; Total Carbohydrates 130g; Sugar 7g; Total Fat 11g; Saturated Fat 2g; Sodium 796mg; Protein 22g; Fiber 7g

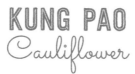

KUNG PAO
Cauliflower

SERVES 4 ∘ PREP TIME: 10 MINUTES ∘ COOK TIME: 25 MINUTES

VEGAN

1 head cauliflower,
 broken into florets
3 tablespoons canola oil
1 teaspoon minced
 peeled fresh ginger
1 teaspoon minced garlic
⅛ teaspoon red
 pepper flakes
Sea salt
Freshly ground
 black pepper
2 tablespoons gluten-free
 soy sauce
2 tablespoons
 balsamic vinegar
1 tablespoon brown sugar
1 cup toasted cashews
4 scallions, white and
 green parts, thinly
 sliced on the bias

Serve this flavorful roasted cauliflower alongside the Hoisin-Glazed Tofu and Green Beans (page 182) with steamed rice for a complete vegan meal. I'm just waiting for the day when someone finally decides to create gluten-free fortune cookies. As much as I love cooking, I'm just not going to make them at home. Plus, you can't write your own fortune!

1. Preheat the oven to 425°F.

2. In a large bowl, toss the cauliflower with the canola oil to coat.

3. Add the ginger, garlic, and red pepper flakes. Season with salt and pepper and toss again.

4. Spread the cauliflower onto a rimmed baking sheet and roast for 20 minutes.

5. Meanwhile, in a small bowl, whisk the soy sauce, vinegar, and brown sugar. Pour this mixture over the cauliflower and roast for 5 minutes more.

6. Toss with the cashews and scallions, and serve hot over rice.

INGREDIENT TIP Chinese black vinegar is a traditional ingredient in kung pao sauce, but it is made with malt, which contains gluten. We substitute wine-based balsamic vinegar here.

PER SERVING Calories 349; Total Carbohydrates 24g; Sugar 8g; Total Fat 27g; Saturated Fat 4g; Sodium 564mg; Protein 7g; Fiber 5g

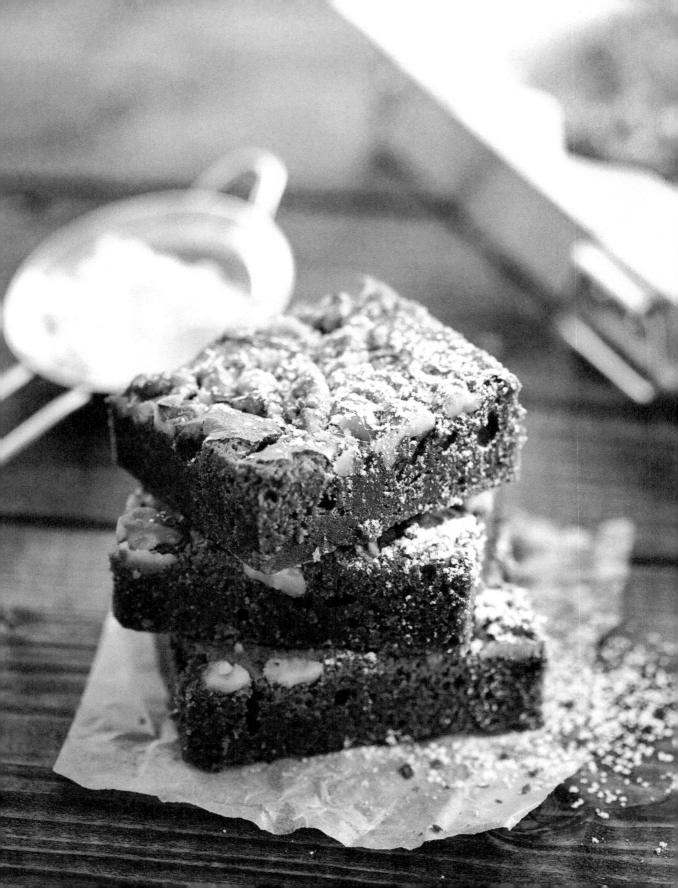

CHAPTER *Eight*

SNACKS AND DESSERTS

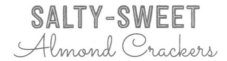

SALTY-SWEET
Almond Crackers

VEGAN

2 cups finely ground
  blanched almond flour
¾ teaspoon sea salt
2 teaspoons sugar
1 tablespoon extra-virgin
  olive oil
1 to 2 tablespoons
  ice-cold water

These naturally gluten-free crackers have a little more heft than traditional grain-based crackers. They're delicious plain or topped with cream cheese and jalapeño jelly, chicken liver pâté, or just a sprinkle of cinnamon and sugar.

1. Preheat the oven to 325°F.

2. In a medium bowl, mix the almond flour, salt, and sugar.

3. Add the olive oil and 1 tablespoon of the cold water. Stir to combine, adding more water as needed until the mixture comes together in a ball.

4. Place the dough onto a sheet of parchment paper and shape it into a rectangle. Top with another sheet of parchment. With a rolling pin, roll the dough to about ⅛ inch thick. Remove the top sheet of parchment. Transfer the dough and parchment to a rimmed baking sheet. Cut the dough into 24 squares. Separate them slightly.

5. Bake for 10 to 12 minutes, checking frequently so they do not burn.

6. Cool completely before storing in an airtight container at room temperature for up to 3 days.

SUBSTITUTION For a garlic and herb cracker, swap the sugar for ½ teaspoon garlic powder and add 1 tablespoon minced fresh herbs, such as basil, parsley, thyme, or rosemary.

PER SERVING Calories 156; Total Carbohydrates 6g; Sugar 2g; Total Fat 14g; Saturated Fat 1g; Sodium 176mg; Protein 5g; Fiber 3g

CHEX PARTY MIX

MAKES 8 CUPS ∘ PREP TIME: 5 MINUTES ∘ COOK TIME: 25 MINUTES

EGG-FREE
MAKE DAIRY-FREE
MAKE VEGAN

2 cups Corn Chex
2 cups Rice Chex
2 cups mixed nuts
1 cup gluten-free pretzels
1 cup bite-size gluten-free
  bagel chips
½ cup (1 stick)
  melted butter
2 garlic cloves, minced
1 teaspoon minced fresh
  herbs, such as parsley,
  basil, or oregano
2 teaspoons gluten-free
  Worcestershire sauce
½ teaspoon sea salt
Pinch cayenne
  pepper (optional)

The premade party mix you buy in stores contains gluten. When you mix your own, not only do you lose the wheat, you can also enjoy a much more flavorful snack.

1. Preheat the oven to 350°F.

2. In a large bowl, combine the Corn Chex, Rice Chex, nuts, pretzels, and bagel chips.

3. In small bowl, stir together the butter, garlic, herbs, Worcestershire sauce, salt, and cayenne pepper (if using).

4. Pour the butter mixture over the cereal and nuts and stir to coat.

5. Spread the mixture on a rimmed baking sheet and bake for 10 minutes. Stir and bake for 10 minutes more. Stir and bake for another 5 minutes, or until the mixture begins to brown.

6. Cool completely before storing in an airtight container at room temperature.

INGREDIENT TIP If you have trouble finding bite-size gluten-free bagel chips, buy the larger size and break them into bite-size pieces before mixing with the other ingredients.

SUBSTITUTION TIP To make this dairy-free and vegan, use canola oil instead of butter.

PER SERVING Calories 215; Total Carbohydrates 15g; Sugar 2g; Total Fat 16g; Saturated Fat 5g; Sodium 286mg; Protein; Fiber 2g

DATE CARAMEL
and Apples

SERVES 4 ° PREP TIME: 20 MINUTES

ALLERGEN-FREE
NUT-FREE
ONE POT
VEGAN

½ cup pitted
  Medjool dates
¼ to ⅓ cup hot water
3 tablespoons coconut
  oil, melted
1 teaspoon vanilla extract
⅛ teaspoon sea salt
2 tart apples, such as
  Granny Smith, cored
  and cut into wedges

The first time I tasted date caramel, I was undone. It requires no cooking and no added sugars, and yet it's sweet, syrupy, and exquisite drizzled over pancakes or used as a dip for apples. Store it in a sealable container for an energizing snack.

1. In a medium heatproof container, combine the dates with sufficient hot water to cover. Soak for 15 minutes.

2. Add the coconut oil, vanilla, and salt. With an immersion blender or standard blender, purée until very smooth.

3. Serve the date caramel with the apple slices.

SERVING TIP If you're packing this treat in a school lunch box, sprinkle the apple slices with lemon juice to keep them from browning and seal in a zip-top bag.

PER SERVING Calories 201; Total Carbohydrates 29g; Sugar 24g; Total Fat 10g; Saturated Fat 9g; Sodium 60mg; Protein 2g; Fiber 4g

TRAIL MIX

MAKES 7½ CUPS ∘ PREP TIME: 5 MINUTES

ONE POT
VEGAN

2 cups almonds
1 cup walnut pieces
1 cup cashews
1 cup shelled
  sunflower seeds
2 cups raisins
½ cup dark chocolate
  chips (optional)

Okay, I'll admit it. I am *that* mom who reads all ingredient labels—even healthy foods, such as trail mix—and puts them back on the shelf if they have too much sugar, or worse, high-fructose corn syrup. That is, unfortunately, the case with many commercial trail mixes, which are heavy on the dried cranberries or chocolate candies. Fortunately, making my own trail mix is a cinch and I get to decide whether and how much of those sweet things to add.

1. In a large bowl, mix the almonds, walnuts, cashews, sunflower seeds, raisins, and chocolate chips (if using).

2. Store in a covered container at room temperature.

INGREDIENT TIP Make your own version of this trail mix with whatever nuts and dried fruit you have on hand. If using the chocolate chips, read the label to ensure they're dairy-free.

PER SERVING Calories 253; Total Carbohydrates 22g; Sugar 13g; Total Fat 17g; Saturated Fat 2g; Sodium 4mg; Protein 7g; Fiber 3g

GRANOLA BARS

MAKES 8 (4-BY-2-INCH) BARS ∘ PREP TIME: 5 MINUTES
COOK TIME: 20 TO 25 MINUTES

DAIRY-FREE
EGG-FREE
VEGETARIAN

3 tablespoons canola oil, divided

2 cups gluten-free rolled oats

½ cup toasted shelled sunflower seeds

½ cup toasted sliced almonds

1 cup raisins, or other dried fruit

¼ cup flax meal

1 teaspoon ground cinnamon

¾ cup honey

½ teaspoon sea salt

1 teaspoon vanilla extract

Most commercial granola bars contain lots of sugar, and conventional oats, which may contain gluten. Homemade versions are similar and often call for wheat germ. This version uses gluten-free oats and flax meal, and gets its sweetness from honey and dried fruit.

1. Preheat the oven to 325°F.

2. Coat the inside of an 8-by-8-inch baking dish with 1 tablespoon of the canola oil.

3. In a large bowl, combine the oats, sunflower seeds, almonds, raisins, flax meal, and cinnamon.

4. In a glass liquid measuring cup, stir together the honey, the remaining 2 tablespoons canola oil, salt, and vanilla. Heat in a microwave oven for 1½ minutes on high. Stir to mix and pour over the oat mixture. Use a spatula to combine the mixture thoroughly.

5. Spread the oat mixture in the prepared pan, pressing down on it with a sheet of parchment paper or your fingers and palms coated with oil.

6. Bake for 20 to 25 minutes until gently browned. Cool and cut into bars.

COOKING TIP For a delicious toasted flavor, spread the oats on a baking sheet and bake for 10 minutes before mixing with the other ingredients.

PER SERVING Calories 347; Total Carbohydrates 58g; Sugar 38g; Total Fat 12g; Saturated Fat 1g; Sodium 123g; Protein 6g; Fiber 5g

CHOCOLATE ALMOND BUTTER CUPS

MAKES 12 CUPS ° PREP TIME: 5 MINUTES ° CHILL TIME: 20 MINUTES

VEGAN

½ cup coconut oil, melted
½ cup creamy
 almond butter
¼ cup maple syrup
½ cup unsweetened
 cocoa powder
½ teaspoon sea salt

I totally understand if you cannot wait the 20 minutes for these delicious treats to chill. May I suggest distraction? Take a walk for 10 minutes in one direction, then you'll have at least a 10-minute walk home. They're still delicious if not thoroughly chilled, but they're absolutely divine when the coconut oil has had a chance to harden fully.

1. Line a 12-cup muffin tin with paper liners.

2. In a blender, or a cup fitted for an immersion blender, combine the coconut oil, almond butter, maple syrup, cocoa powder, and salt. Purée until smooth.

3. Pour about 2 to 3 tablespoons of the mixture into each muffin cup. Refrigerate for at least 20 minutes until set. Keep refrigerated.

SERVING TIP If packing this treat for a school lunch, pack it in a covered container next to an ice pack to keep it cool.

PER SERVING Calories 170; Total Carbohydrates 8g; Sugar 4g; Total Fat 16g; Saturated Fat 9g; Sodium 79mg; Protein 3g; Fiber 2g

COOKIE DOUGH
Date Bars

MAKES 16 BARS ° PREP TIME: 5 MINUTES

VEGAN

1 cup pitted Medjool dates
1 ½ cups walnuts
¼ teaspoon sea salt
1 cup dark chocolate
  pieces, at least
  70 percent cacao

Homemade versions of the popular Lärabars abound and all have a very similar ratio of ingredients, 1 part pitted dates to 1 to 1 ½ parts nuts. This is one of my favorites and reminds me of chocolate chip cookie dough.

1. In a food processor, combine the dates, walnuts, and salt. Pulse until coarsely ground. You should easily be able to pinch the dough between your fingers and have it stick together.

2. Remove the processor blade and stir in the chocolate pieces. Transfer the dough to a work surface. Firmly press the dough into a rectangular shape, about 8 inches by 5 inches. Slice into 16 bars and refrigerate, covered.

INGREDIENT TIP To ensure your chocolate is dairy-free, read the label.

SUBSTITUTION TIP Let your imagination guide you to new flavor combinations. I enjoy swapping blanched almonds for walnuts and adding 1 cup dried cherries.

PER SERVING Calories 160; Total Carbohydrates 16g; Sugar 13g; Total Fat 10g; Saturated Fat 3g; Sodium 40mg; Protein 4g; Fiber 2g

FIG BARS

MAKES 9 BARS ∘ PREP TIME: 10 MINUTES ∘ COOK TIME: 20 MINUTES

DAIRY-FREE
VEGETARIAN

1 cup finely ground
blanched almond flour

¼ cup coconut flour

¼ cup tapioca
flour (starch)

½ teaspoon sea salt

¼ cup palm
shortening, melted

1 egg

¼ cup plus 1 tablespoon
maple syrup, divided

1 ½ cups dried figs,
stemmed

1 tablespoon freshly
squeezed lemon juice

¼ teaspoon ground
cinnamon

These healthy fig bars contain less sugar than packaged fig cookies. Instead of the traditional sandwich-style bar, I decided to make it easy and simply sprinkle the topping over the filling. If you prefer, roll out the remaining crust layer and press it onto the top.

1. Preheat the oven to 350°F.

2. Line an 8-by-8-inch baking dish with parchment paper.

3. In a food processor, combine the almond flour, coconut flour, tapioca flour, and salt.

4. Add the palm shortening, egg, and 1 tablespoon of the maple syrup. Pulse until just blended.

5. Transfer half of the crust mixture to the prepared pan and press it down into the pan with your fingers. Put the remaining crust mixture into a small bowl. Remove the processor blade and wipe out the processor bowl with a paper towel.

6. In the food processor, put the figs, the remaining ¼ cup maple syrup, lemon juice, and cinnamon. Blend until mostly smooth. Carefully spread this mixture over the crust layer.

7. Sprinkle the remaining crust pieces over the top. Bake for 20 minutes until the top is gently browned.

SUBSTITUTION TIP You can also use brown sugar in place of the maple syrup. Add 2 tablespoons of water to the filling to compensate for the lost liquid.

PER SERVING Calories 238; Total Carbohydrates 31g; Sugar 23g; Total Fat 13g; Saturated Fat 3g; Sodium 117mg; Protein 4g; Fiber 5g

APPLE FRITTERS

MAKES 8 FRITTERS ° PREP TIME: 10 MINUTES ° COOK TIME: 14 MINUTES

EGG-FREE
NUT-FREE
MAKE ALLERGEN-FREE
MAKE DAIRY-FREE
MAKE VEGAN

½ cup garbanzo bean (chickpea) flour
½ cup plus 2 tablespoons powdered sugar, divided
2 teaspoons aluminum-free, double-acting baking powder
2 teaspoons ground cinnamon
½ teaspoon ground nutmeg
¼ teaspoon sea salt
3 apples, peeled, cored, and diced (about 1½ cups)
½ cup plus 2 tablespoons milk, divided
Canola oil, for frying

These easy apple fritters capture the flavors of the original deep-fried donut, but only require a fraction of the time—and you skip the deep-fry for a simple panfry-and-steam technique.

1. Into a large bowl, sift the garbanzo bean flour, ½ cup of the powdered sugar, the baking powder, cinnamon, nutmeg, and salt.

2. Stir in the apples.

3. Whisk in ½ cup of the milk until no lumps remain.

4. In a large skillet or sauté pan over medium-high heat, heat about ½ inch of the oil until hot, 1 to 2 minutes. Do not leave the pan unattended!

5. Scoop about ½ cup fritter batter into the hot oil to make one fritter. Repeat with the remaining batter. You will need to do this in two batches so as not to crowd the pan. Cook for 3 minutes, then place a lid on the pan to continue cooking 2 to 3 minutes more until the top is set. Transfer the cooked fritters to a cooling rack and allow the oil to heat up again before using the remaining batter.

6. In a small bowl, whisk the remaining 2 tablespoons powdered sugar with the remaining 2 tablespoons of the milk. Drizzle this glaze over the cooked fritters.

SUBSTITUTION TIP To make this dairy-free, allergen-free, and vegan, use a nondairy milk such as rice milk.

PER SERVING Calories 148; Total Carbohydrates 25g; Sugar 15g; Total Fat 5g; Saturated Fat 1g; Sodium 72mg; Protein 3g; Fiber 4g

NO-BAKE CHERRY CHEESECAKE

SERVES 9 ° PREP TIME: 5 MINUTES ° CHILL TIME: 25 MINUTES

EGG-FREE
NUT-FREE
VEGETARIAN

2 cups gluten-free pretzels
1 tablespoon brown sugar
½ cup (1 stick) melted
  unsalted butter
2 (8-ounce) packages
  cream cheese, at
  room temperature
1 cup sour cream
1 cup powdered sugar
1 teaspoon vanilla extract
1 (15-ounce) can gluten-
  free cherry pie filling

My mom made this for my brothers' and my birthdays for several years. The cloying sweetness of the cherry pie filling, offset by the creamy tartness of the cheesecake layer and the salty graham cracker crust, was, as far as we were concerned, even better than growing a year older. This version uses salty gluten-free pretzels and a scant amount of brown sugar for a more savory crust.

1. In a food processor, pulse the pretzels and brown sugar until finely ground. Add the butter and pulse until just integrated.

2. Pour the pretzel mixture into an 8-by-8-inch baking dish and press down with a fork. Put in the freezer for 5 minutes.

3. In a large bowl, use a hand mixer to whip the cream cheese, sour cream, powdered sugar, and vanilla until smooth. Carefully spread this mixture over the chilled crust. Return to the freezer for 15 minutes more.

4. Gently spread the cherry pie filling over the cheesecake layer to cover. Refrigerate until ready to serve, at least 10 minutes.

INGREDIENT TIP Look for a cherry pie filling without high fructose corn syrup, such as Baker Naturals Cherry Pie Filling.

PER SERVING Calories 474; Total Carbohydrates 39g; Sugar 15g; Total Fat 34g; Saturated Fat 21g; Sodium 395mg; Protein 6g; Fiber 1g

CHOCOLATE CHIP COOKIES

MAKES 36 COOKIES ° PREP TIME: 5 MINUTES ° COOK TIME: 9 MINUTES

DAIRY-FREE
NUT-FREE
VEGETARIAN

1 cup shortening

¾ cup packed
 brown sugar

½ cup granulated sugar

1 tablespoon vanilla
 extract

2 eggs

1 teaspoon sea salt

2 cups Whole-Grain
 Gluten-Free Flour
 Blend (page 25)

¼ cup cornstarch

1 teaspoon baking soda

2 cups dark
 chocolate chips

I won my husband's attention in college with my family recipe for chocolate chip cookies. So, when it came time to craft a gluten-free version, the expectations were high. Fortunately, these come pretty darn close.

1. Preheat the oven to 350°F.

2. Line 2 rimmed baking sheets with parchment paper.

3. In a large bowl and with a hand mixer, cream the shortening, brown sugar, and granulated sugar until fluffy, about 1 minute.

4. Add the vanilla, eggs, and salt and beat until thoroughly emulsified, about 1 minute.

5. Sift in the flour blend, cornstarch, and baking soda. Mix thoroughly.

6. Fold in the chocolate chips.

7. For each cookie, spoon about 2 heaping tablespoons of dough onto the prepared sheets, leaving 2 inches between cookies; they will spread.

8. Bake for about 9 minutes until gently browned and barely set in the middle. Cool for 1 minute before transferring to a cooling rack to cool completely.

INGREDIENT TIP Regarding the chocolate chips, read the label to ensure yours are dairy-free.

PER SERVING Calories 155; Total Carbohydrates 18g; Sugar 11g; Total Fat 9g; Saturated Fat 4g; Sodium 98mg; Protein 2g; Fiber 1g

COCONUT MACAROONS

MAKES 24 MACAROONS ∘ PREP TIME: 5 MINUTES ∘ COOK TIME: 20 MINUTES

DAIRY-FREE
NUT-FREE
VEGETARIAN

2 egg whites
Pinch sea salt
¼ cup sugar
1 teaspoon vanilla extract
2 cups unsweetened
   shredded coconut

These coconut macaroons are a cinch to make. Plus they're bound by unsweetened coconut, which is rich in fiber, healthy fats, protein, and micronutrients.

1. Preheat the oven to 325°F.

2. Line a rimmed baking sheet with parchment paper.

3. In a medium bowl with a hand mixer, beat the egg whites and salt until soft peaks form.

4. Beat in the sugar 1 tablespoon at a time until the egg whites are thick and glossy, about 1 minute.

5. Whisk in the vanilla.

6. Fold in the coconut until just integrated.

7. Using a 1-tablespoon measuring spoon or an ice cream scoop, scoop the batter and gently drop the portions onto the prepared baking sheet in neat mounds.

8. Bake for 20 minutes, or until barely beginning to brown. Cool before eating or storing.

SERVING TIP Melt ½ cup of dark chocolate chips in a double boiler or thick-bottomed skillet and dip the bottoms of the cooled macaroons into the melted chocolate. Place on a clean sheet of parchment to harden. Store in the refrigerator.

INGREDIENT TIP To ensure your chocolate chips are dairy-free, read the label.

PER SERVING Calories 33; Total Carbohydrates 4g; Sugar 3g; Total Fat 2g; Saturated Fat 2g; Sodium 16mg; Protein 1g; Fiber 1g

BROWNIES

SERVES 10 ° PREP TIME: 5 MINUTES ° COOK TIME: 20 TO 22 MINUTES

VEGETARIAN
MAKE DAIRY-FREE
MAKE NUT-FREE

½ cup (1 stick) butter,
plus more for coating
the pan
1 tablespoon unsweetened
cocoa powder
1 (11-ounce) bag dark
chocolate chips,
60 percent cacao
or more, divided
4 eggs
½ cup packed
brown sugar
1 tablespoon vanilla
extract
½ teaspoon sea salt
1 cup Whole-Grain
Gluten-Free Flour
Blend (page 25)
1 cup walnut pieces
(optional)

Brownies should never *need* frosting. They should be crisp around the edges with a light crust on the top and densely fudgy inside. They should be so decadent and decidedly not cake that you don't want anything else, except perhaps another brownie. Then again, if you *want* frosting, who am I to stop you?

1. Preheat the oven to 350°F.

2. Coat the inside of a 9-by-13 baking pan with butter.

3. Add the cocoa powder and gently shake the pan to disburse the cocoa. Discard the leftover cocoa.

4. In a double boiler or thick-bottomed skillet, melt the remaining ½ cup butter and 1 cup of the chocolate chips. Let cool.

5. In a large bowl with a hand mixer, beat the eggs, brown sugar, vanilla, and salt for 1 minute until smooth.

6. Add the melted and cooled chocolate. Beat until just integrated.

7. Sift in the flour blend and stir until just integrated. Fold in the remaining chocolate chips.

8. Spread the batter into the prepared pan, top with the walnut pieces (if using), and bake for 20 to 22 minutes until crisp around the edges and just set in the middle. Cool and cut into bars.

INGREDIENT TIP Ghirardelli makes a dark chocolate chip with 60 percent cacao that I recommend for this recipe.

COOKING TIP No, it's not a typo—there is no leavening needed for brownies beyond the eggs.

SERVING TIP For a pretty presentation, sprinkle 1 to 2 tablespoons of powdered sugar or unsweetened cocoa powder over the brownies.

SUBSTITUTION TIP To make this dairy-free, use shortening in place of the butter and make sure the chocolate chips are dairy-free.

PER SERVING Calories 351; Total Carbohydrates 36g; Sugar 23g; Total Fat 20g; Saturated Fat 13g; Sodium 211mg; Protein 6g; Fiber 2g

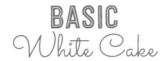

BASIC
White Cake

NUT-FREE
VEGETARIAN
MAKE DAIRY-FREE

½ cup (1 stick) plus
 1 tablespoon butter
1¾ cups plus 2 teaspoons
 Whole-Grain Gluten-Free
 Flour Blend (page 25)
2 teaspoons aluminum-
 free, double-acting
 baking powder
¼ teaspoon sea salt
¾ cup sugar
½ cup milk
1 teaspoon vanilla extract
4 egg whites
¼ teaspoon cream
 of tartar

Ready for some good news? Cakes are best when made with a low-gluten flour known as cake flour. And so gluten-free flour blends are especially well suited to the job. Take this cake in whatever direction you like. Fill it with strawberry preserves or lime curd, or use it to make a Boston cream pie or an extra-special birthday cake.

1. Preheat the oven to 375°F.

2. Use 1 tablespoon of the butter to coat the inside of two 8-inch cake pans. Line the bottoms with parchment paper.

3. In a medium bowl, sift together the flour blend, baking powder, and salt.

4. In a large bowl, whip the remaining ½ cup butter and the sugar until light and fluffy.

5. To the butter and sugar mixture, add the milk, vanilla, and the flour mixture and beat until smooth. Do not overmix.

6. In a clean, dry, large bowl, using clean beaters, whip the egg whites and cream of tartar until stiff peaks form.

7. Fold ⅓ of the egg whites into the batter to lighten it. Then fold in the remaining egg whites, folding just until combined.

8. Pour the batter into the prepared pans. Bake for 20 minutes, or until a cake tester poked into the center comes out clean. Cool the cakes before removing them from the pans.

INGREDIENT TIP Cream of tartar may not seem like it matters, but it helps the egg whites maintain their volume and withstand the heat of cooking.

SUBSTITUTION TIP To make this cake dairy-free, use canola oil in place of the butter.

PER SERVING Calories 304; Total Carbohydrates 41g; Sugar 20g; Total Fat 14g; Saturated Fat 8g; Sodium 176mg; Protein 5g; Fiber 1g

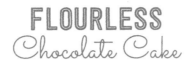

FLOURLESS
Chocolate Cake

SERVES 6 ∘ PREP TIME: 5 MINUTES ∘ COOK TIME: 25 MINUTES

NUT-FREE
VEGETARIAN

½ cup (1 stick) plus
  1 tablespoon butter
3½ ounces dark
  chocolate, at least
  70 percent cacao
3 eggs
½ cup packed
  brown sugar
¼ teaspoon sea salt
½ cup plus 2 tablespoons
  unsweetened
  cocoa powder

This flourless chocolate cake has a rich, dark chocolaty flavor. It is delicious served with a dollop of whipped cream or crème fraîche.

1. Preheat the oven to 375°F.

2. Coat the inside of an 8-inch cake pan with 1 tablespoon of the butter and line the bottom with a piece of parchment paper.

3. In a double boiler or a thick-bottomed skillet, melt the remaining ½ cup butter and the dark chocolate. Cool.

4. In a medium bowl, whisk the eggs, brown sugar, and salt.

5. Stir in the melted chocolate and butter until thoroughly integrated.

6. Sift in ½ cup of the cocoa powder and whisk until thoroughly mixed.

7. Pour the batter into the prepared pan and bake for 25 minutes. Let cool for 10 minutes and then transfer from the cake pan to a serving plate.

8. Let cool to room temperature. Sift the remaining 2 tablespoons cocoa powder over the top.

COOKING TIP If you have a springform pan, use it with this recipe and easily remove the sides for serving.

PER SERVING Calories 339; Total Carbohydrates 27g; Sugar 21g; Total Fat 26g; Saturated Fat 16g; Sodium 250mg; Protein 6g; Fiber 3g

BLACKBERRY AND BLUEBERRY
Crumble

SERVES 6 ∘ PREP TIME: 5 MINUTES ∘ COOK TIME: 25 MINUTES

EGG-FREE
NUT-FREE
MAKE ALLERGEN-FREE
MAKE DAIRY-FREE
MAKE VEGAN

5 tablespoons
  butter, divided
4 cups fresh blackberries
2 cups fresh blueberries
6 tablespoons
  sugar, divided
3 tablespoons tapioca
  flour (starch)
1 cup Whole-Grain
  Gluten-Free Flour
  Blend (page 25)
¼ teaspoon sea salt

Every summer when the Oregon blackberries ripened, my family and I would pick them for the local restaurants. In the process, we stained ourselves purple and developed a deep discernment for what the ripest berries look and taste like. Of course, we always brought some home and, after eating our fill, made pies and other desserts. This one is super easy to throw together before dinner so it has time to cool after baking.

1. Preheat the oven to 350°F.

2. Coat the inside of a 2-quart casserole dish with 1 tablespoon of butter.

3. Add the blackberries and blueberries to the prepared dish and top with 2 tablespoons of the sugar and the tapioca flour. Gently toss to mix.

4. In a medium bowl, combine the remaining 4 tablespoons butter, remaining 4 tablespoons sugar, the flour blend, and salt. Mix with a spatula or your clean hands and then crumble it over the berries.

5. Bake for 25 minutes, or until the top is golden brown and the berries are bubbling. Cool briefly before serving.

SUBSTITUTION TIP To make this allergen-free, dairy-free, and vegan, use palm shortening or another nondairy butter substitute in place of the butter.

PER SERVING Calories 290; Total Carbohydrates 48g; Sugar 22g; Total Fat 10g; Saturated Fat 6g; Sodium 148mg; Protein 4g; Fiber 7g

CARROT CAKE

SERVES 8 ° PREP TIME: 10 MINUTES ° COOK TIME: 20 MINUTES

VEGETARIAN

MAKE NUT-FREE

1 tablespoon shortening

1 ½ cups Whole-Grain Gluten-Free Flour Blend (page 25)

1 teaspoon baking soda

1 teaspoon ground cinnamon

½ teaspoon freshly grated nutmeg

½ teaspoon sea salt

2 eggs

½ cup packed brown sugar

⅓ cup canola oil

3 carrots, shredded

½ cup raisins (optional)

¼ cup finely chopped walnuts (optional)

1 (8-ounce) package cream cheese, at room temperature

2 cups powdered sugar

1 teaspoon vanilla extract

Cream cheese frosting was always my favorite part of carrot cake while growing up. It took me until adulthood to appreciate the delicate spices and intense carrot taste of this cake. Use organic carrots, which have a more mellow flavor than conventionally grown carrots.

1. Preheat the oven to 350°F.

2. Coat the inside of an 8-inch cake pan with the shortening.

3. In a large bowl, whisk the flour blend, baking soda, cinnamon, nutmeg, and salt.

4. In a medium bowl, whisk the eggs, brown sugar, and canola oil. Add the egg mixture to the flour mixture and stir together until just combined.

5. Fold in the carrots, raisins (if using), and walnuts (if using).

6. Pour the batter into the prepared pan. Bake for 20 minutes, or until a cake tester poked into the center comes out clean.

7. Meanwhile, in a medium bowl and using a hand mixer, combine the cream cheese, powdered sugar, and vanilla. Whip until smooth and fluffy.

8. Cool the cake before frosting.

COOKING TIP You can also pour this batter into a muffin tin lined with paper cups to make individual carrot cupcakes.

PER SERVING Calories 457; Total Carbohydrates 60g; Sugar 40g; Total Fat 22g; Saturated Fat 8g; Sodium 394mg; Protein; Fiber 1g

CHOCOLATE-ZUCCHINI CAKE

SERVES 8 ° PREP TIME: 10 MINUTES ° COOK TIME: 20 TO 25 MINUTES

VEGETARIAN
MAKE DAIRY-FREE

5 tablespoons
  butter, at room
  temperature, divided
½ cup packed
  brown sugar
4 eggs
1 tablespoon vanilla
  extract
1 cup finely ground
  blanched almond flour
1 tablespoon coconut flour
½ cup unsweetened
  cocoa powder
1 teaspoon baking soda
½ teaspoon sea salt
1 medium zucchini,
  shredded (about
  1 loosely packed cup)

Zucchini virtually disappears into the rich, chocolate batter, leaving a light, moist cake with extra fiber and nutrients. But, shhh, let's not tell the kids, shall we?

1. Preheat the oven to 325°F.

2. Coat the inside of a 9-inch cake pan with 1 tablespoon of butter. Line the pan with parchment paper.

3. In a large mixing bowl, use a hand mixer to beat the brown sugar and remaining 4 tablespoons butter for about 1 minute.

4. Add the eggs and vanilla, and beat for about 1 minute until smooth.

5. Sift in the almond flour, coconut flour, cocoa powder, baking soda, and salt. Stir until integrated.

6. With your hands, squeeze the excess moisture from the zucchini and then fold it into the cake batter.

7. Pour the batter into the prepared pan. Bake for 20 to 25 minutes, or until a cake tester comes out clean. Cool 10 minutes before removing from the pan to cool on a rack.

INGREDIENT TIP The quality of your cocoa powder really does make a difference. It's worth spending a little extra money on one that's good. My favorite brand is Equal Exchange Baking Cocoa, which is grown by small farmer co-ops and is fairly traded.

SUBSTITUTION TIP To make this dairy-free, use shortening or oil in place of the butter.

PER SERVING Calories 219; Total Carbohydrates 16g; Sugar 10g; Total Fat 16g; Saturated Fat 6g; Sodium 364mg; Protein 7g; Fiber 3g

PEACH GALETTE

SERVES 6 ° PREP TIME: 10 MINUTES ° COOK TIME: 15 MINUTES

VEGETARIAN
MAKE DAIRY-FREE

1 ½ cups finely ground
  blanched almond flour
2 tablespoons tapioca
  flour (starch)
¼ teaspoon sea salt
1 egg, whisked, divided
3 tablespoons cold butter
2 to 5 teaspoons
  ice-cold water
6 to 8 small peaches,
  pitted, peeled, and
  thinly sliced
1 teaspoon sugar

During our first summer in Santa Barbara, some people from church invited us to pick peaches from their tree while they were away on vacation. The kids helped me, even climbing into the tree to carefully select the ripest fruits. There were so many—we grilled them, dried them, made cobbler, and crafted this rustic summer tart. It's naturally sweet and delicious, but if your peaches aren't the ripest, sprinkle the top with a tablespoon or two of brown sugar.

1. Preheat the oven to 400°F.

2. In a food processor, combine the almond flour, tapioca flour, and salt. Pulse a few times to mix.

3. Transfer 1 tablespoon of the whisked egg to a small cup and set aside. Add the remaining egg, and the butter to the processor. Blend for a few seconds, just until integrated.

4. Add 1 to 2 teaspoons of the cold water and blend just until the dough forms a ball.

5. Transfer the dough to a sheet of parchment paper on the work surface. Place another piece of parchment over the top, and use a rolling pin to flatten the dough into a 10-inch circle. Remove the top sheet of parchment paper.

6. Arrange the peach slices in a circular pattern in the center of the tart. Fold the edges of the crust over the peaches and pleat extra all the way around.

7. Mix the reserved egg with the remaining 1 tablespoon cold water and brush the crust with it.

8. Sprinkle the sugar over the crust.

9. Bake for 15 minutes, or until the peaches are soft and the crust is browned.

SUBSTITUTION TIP This recipe is good with a variety of soft fruits, such as plums, blackberries, strawberries, or mango.

SUBSTITUTION TIP To make this dairy-free, use palm shortening in place of the butter.

PER SERVING Calories 262; Total Carbohydrates 21g; Sugar 13g; Total Fat 19g; Saturated Fat 5g; Sodium 130mg; Protein 7g; Fiber 5g

CHOCOLATE MOUSSE

SERVES 4 ° PREP TIME: 5 MINUTES PLUS 20 MINUTES CHILLING TIME
COOK TIME: 3 MINUTES

NUT-FREE
VEGETARIAN
MAKE ALLERGEN-FREE
MAKE DAIRY-FREE

3½ ounces dark
  chocolate, at least
  70 percent cacao
2 tablespoons butter
4 eggs, separated
1 teaspoon vanilla extract
2 tablespoons sugar
⅛ teaspoon sea salt

When it comes to chocolate mousse, I want the intense, chocolaty flavor of my favorite dark chocolate—70 percent cacao Valrhona chocolate—but I want it to last longer than the small square I usually enjoy. This chocolate mousse delivers!

1. In a double boiler or a thick-bottomed skillet over low heat, melt the chocolate and butter. Set aside to cool slightly.

2. When the chocolate is cool, whisk 3 egg yolks into it, one at a time, along with the vanilla. Save the remaining egg yolk for another use.

3. In a large bowl, whip the egg whites until soft peaks form. Add the salt and 1 tablespoon of sugar at a time. Continue beating until stiff peaks form.

4. Fold one-third of the egg whites into the chocolate mixture to lighten it. Add the remaining egg whites and fold gently just until combined. Be careful not to deflate the mixture with vigorous stirring.

5. Evenly divide the mousse among 4 small serving cups and chill for at least 20 minutes. You can make this several hours in advance, if you wish.

COOKING TIP Consuming raw eggs poses a risk of salmonella, a foodborne illness. Pasteurized eggs reduce this risk, but do not whip up as easily.

SUBSTITUTION TIP To make this allergen-free and dairy-free, use a nondairy butter and ensure that the chocolate chips are dairy-free.

PER SERVING Calories 272; Total Carbohydrates 21g; Sugar 19g; Total Fat 18g; Saturated Fat 10g; Sodium 181mg; Protein 8g; Fiber 1g

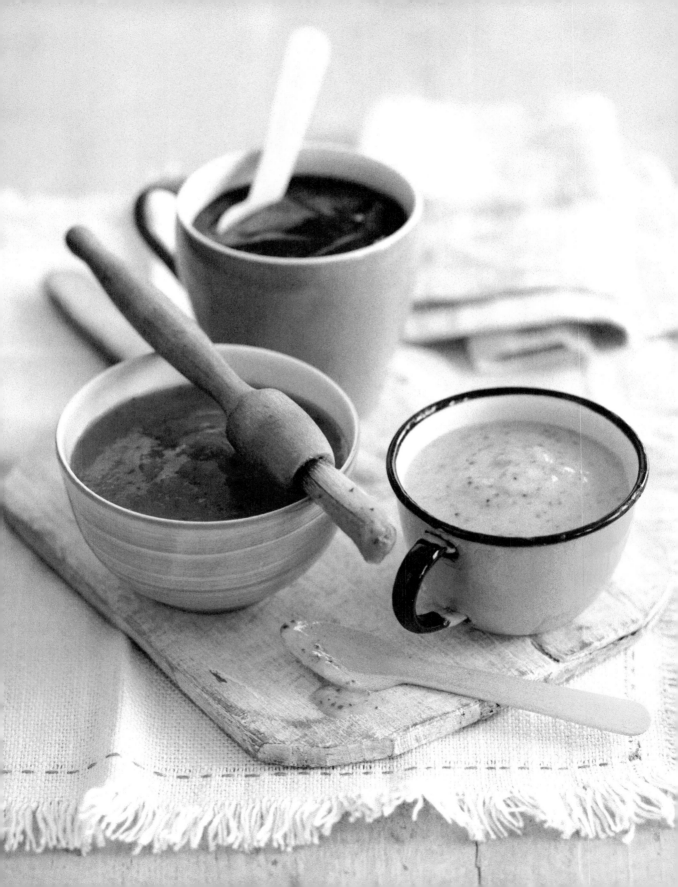

CHAPTER
Nine

SAUCES, CONDIMENTS, AND DRESSINGS

CHICKEN STOCK

MAKES 1½ QUARTS ∘ PREP TIME: 1 MINUTE
COOK TIME: 25 MINUTES, OR LONGER AS TIME ALLOWS

ALLERGEN-FREE
DAIRY-FREE
EGG-FREE
NUT-FREE
ONE POT
SLOW COOKER OPTION

1 pound chicken bones
2 quarts water
1 teaspoon apple cider
  vinegar
Sea salt

Some chicken broths contain gluten and other additives that cause reactions in people with celiac disease, wheat allergies, or nonceliac gluten sensitivity. Fortunately, making your own chicken stock is a cinch. Once you start making it, you'll realize it is not an exact science and requires about as much work as boiling water. I like to use the backbone from the Basic Roast Chicken (page 128) as well as the leftover chicken carcass to make this stock.

1. In a large pot over high heat, combine the chicken bones, water, and apple cider vinegar. Season with salt.

2. Bring to a vigorous simmer. Turn down the heat to low and cook for at least 25 minutes, or longer to intensify the flavor.

SLOW COOKER OPTION Place all the ingredients in a slow cooker and cook for 8 hours on low.

PER SERVING (1 CUP) Calories 67; Total Carbohydrates 4g; Sugar 0g; Total Fat 3g; Saturated Fat 1g; Sodium 91mg; Protein 6g; Fiber 0g

GRAVY

MAKES 2 CUPS ∘ PREP TIME: 5 MINUTES ∘ COOK TIME: 4 MINUTES

EGG-FREE
NUT-FREE
ONE POT
MAKE DAIRY-FREE

3 tablespoons roast turkey
   or chicken pan drippings
1 tablespoon butter
3 tablespoons Whole-
   Grain Gluten-Free Flour
   Blend (page 25)
2 cups chicken broth
Sea salt
Freshly ground
   black pepper

No Thanksgiving is complete without gravy, but it is traditionally thickened with wheat flour. This version gets a flavor hit from the turkey pan drippings (you can use chicken drippings instead if that's what you have) and is thickened with a gluten-free flour.

1. In a small saucepan over medium heat, heat the pan drippings and butter until gently simmering.

2. Whisk in the flour blend until no lumps remain. Cook for 2 minutes, or longer for a deeper colored and flavored roux.

3. All at once, add the chicken broth, whisking vigorously. Turn up the heat to medium-high and bring to a simmer. Cook for about 2 minutes, stirring, until thickened.

4. Season with salt and pepper.

INGREDIENT TIP If you're using a stove top–safe roasting pan to cook the turkey or chicken, make the gravy directly in the pan. Use a whisk or wooden spoon to scrape up dark flavorful bits on the bottom of the pan.

SUBSTITUTION TIP To make this dairy-free, use canola oil in place of the butter.

PER SERVING Calories 152; Total Carbohydrates 5g; Sugar 0g; Total Fat 13g; Saturated Fat 5g; Sodium 287mg; Protein 3g; Fiber 0g

WHITE SAUCE

MAKES 2 CUPS ° PREP TIME: 5 MINUTES ° COOK TIME: 4 MINUTES

EGG-FREE
NUT-FREE
ONE POT
VEGETARIAN

3 tablespoons Whole-
Grain Gluten-Free
Flour Blend (page 25)
3 tablespoons butter
2 cups milk
Sea salt
White pepper

Most white sauces begin with a roux made with equal parts butter and flour. The roux is then cooked over low heat for a couple minutes and then milk is whisked in to create a sauce. Alternatively, the roux is allowed to cook for longer and darken into a deep amber, lending it a rich flavor.

1. In a medium saucepan over medium heat, stir together the flour blend and butter. Whisk to remove any lumps. Cook for 2 minutes, or longer for a deeper roux.

2. All at once add the milk, whisking vigorously. Cook for about 2 minutes until thickened. Do not boil.

3. Season with salt and white pepper.

INGREDIENT TIP For convenience, you can use any store-bought whole-grain gluten-free flour blend in place of the flour blend in this book.

VARIATION TIP To make a simple cheese sauce, allow the white sauce to cool for 1 minute and then stir in 1 teaspoon minced garlic and 1 cup of finely grated Cheddar or Parmesan cheese until melted.

PER SERVING (½ CUP) Calories 159; Total Carbohydrates 11g; Sugar 6g; Total Fat 11g; Saturated Fat 7g; Sodium 177mg; Protein 5g; Fiber 0g

BARBECUE SAUCE

MAKES 2 CUPS ∘ PREP TIME: 5 MINUTES ∘ COOK TIME: 12 MINUTES

ALLERGEN-FREE
NUT-FREE
ONE POT
VEGAN

1 tablespoon extra-virgin
 olive oil
1 yellow onion, minced
2 garlic cloves, minced
2 Medjool dates, pitted
 and minced
1 (15-ounce) can
 tomato sauce
2 teaspoons
 smoked paprika
1 teaspoon ground cumin
1 teaspoon Dijon mustard
1 tablespoon
 balsamic vinegar

This is my go-to barbecue sauce because it's flavorful and has no refined sugar or artificial ingredients.

1. In a small saucepan over medium heat, heat the olive oil.

2. Stir in the onion and garlic and cook for about 5 minutes until softened.

3. Add the dates and cook for 2 minutes more, breaking them up with a wooden spoon.

4. Stir in the tomato sauce, paprika, cumin, mustard, and vinegar. Whisk to combine. Simmer gently for 5 minutes. Refrigerate, covered, for up to 3 days.

COOKING TIP Make this sauce even more quickly by swapping the onion and garlic for 1 tablespoon onion powder and ½ teaspoon garlic powder. Swap the dates for 2 tablespoons brown sugar or honey. Whisk to mix thoroughly.

PER SERVING (¼ CUP) Calories 44; Total Carbohydrates 6g; Sugar 4g; Total Fat 2g; Saturated Fat 0g; Sodium 287mg; Protein 1g; Fiber 2g

TACO SEASONING

ALLERGEN-FREE
NUT-FREE
ONE POT
VEGAN

2 tablespoons
 ground cumin
2 tablespoons
 smoked paprika
2 tablespoons ancho
 chile powder
1 teaspoon ground
 oregano
1 teaspoon onion powder
1 teaspoon garlic powder
¼ teaspoon
 cayenne pepper

Packaged taco seasoning is expensive for what you get: spices and fillers such as wheat starch, salt, and sugar. But once I started making my own taco seasoning, I never looked back. Mix up a batch of this and store it in your cupboard to flavor ground beef, black beans, and rice. It's also perfect for chili, spicy soups, and fresh salsa.

1. In a small bowl, mix the cumin, paprika, ancho chile powder, oregano, onion powder, garlic powder, and cayenne pepper.

2. Store in an airtight container at room temperature in a dark pantry.

INGREDIENT TIP For even more flavor, toast whole cumin seeds in a dry skillet for 1 to 2 minutes and then grind them with a mortar and pestle.

PER SERVING (2 TEASPOONS) Calories 13; Total Carbohydrates 2g; Sugar 0g; Total Fat 1g; Saturated Fat 0g; Sodium 15mg; Protein 1g; Fiber 1g

ENCHILADA SAUCE

MAKES 2 CUPS ° PREP TIME: 5 MINUTES ° COOK TIME: 12 MINUTES

ALLERGEN-FREE
NUT-FREE
ONE POT
VEGAN

1 tablespoon extra-virgin
  olive oil
1 yellow onion, minced
4 garlic cloves, minced
1 (15-ounce) can
  tomato sauce
1 tablespoon
  smoked paprika
1 tablespoon
  ground cumin
1 teaspoon ancho
  chile powder
⅛ teaspoon
  cayenne pepper
Sea salt
Freshly ground
  black pepper

Some enchilada sauces are thickened with wheat flour. However, using a thick tomato sauce and skipping the broth yields a naturally thick sauce that's perfect for pouring over gluten-free enchiladas.

1. In a small saucepan over medium heat, heat the olive oil.

2. Add the onion and garlic and cook for about 5 minutes, stirring occasionally, until softened.

3. Stir in the tomato sauce, paprika, cumin, ancho chile powder, and cayenne pepper. Simmer gently for 5 minutes.

4. Season with salt and pepper.

SUBSTITUTION TIP If you've already made a batch of Taco Seasoning (page 216), use 2½ tablespoons of it in place of the other spices (paprika, cumin, ancho chile powder, and cayenne) in this recipe.

PER SERVING (¼ CUP) Calories 42; Total Carbohydrates 6g; Sugar 3g; Total Fat 2g; Saturated Fat 0g; Sodium 315mg; Protein 1g; Fiber 2g

BASIC SALAD
Dressing

MAKES ¾ CUP ° PREP TIME: 5 MINUTES

ALLERGEN-FREE
NUT-FREE
ONE POT
VEGAN

½ cup extra-virgin olive oil
¼ cup red wine vinegar
Sea salt
Freshly ground
  black pepper

It might seem like making your own salad dressing is time consuming, but it takes about as much time as deciphering the dozens of ingredients found in most bottled salad dressings. Bonus: You can adapt the flavors to whatever you're serving. This recipe is the basic formula for a red wine vinaigrette, followed by several variations to get you started making your own dressings.

1. In a small Mason jar, combine the olive oil and vinegar. Season with salt and pepper. Seal the lid and shake the jar to emulsify the ingredients.

2. Refrigerate, covered, for up to 3 days. Bring out and let sit on the counter for 30 minutes to warm the oil before using. Shake again before pouring.

INGREDIENT TIP To reduce the amount of oil in the recipe, add an emulsifier, such as honey or Dijon mustard.

PER SERVING (2 TABLESPOONS) Calories 146; Total Carbohydrates 0g; Sugar 0g; Total Fat 17g; Saturated Fat 2g; Sodium 40mg; Protein 0g; Fiber 0g

WHITE WINE
Vinaigrette

MAKES ¾ CUP ∘ PREP TIME: 5 MINUTES

ALLERGEN-FREE
DAIRY-FREE
EGG-FREE
NUT-FREE
ONE POT
VEGETARIAN
MAKE VEGAN

½ cup extra-virgin olive oil
2 tablespoons white
  wine vinegar
2 tablespoons freshly
  squeezed lemon juice
1 teaspoon minced
  fresh thyme
½ teaspoon Dijon mustard
½ teaspoon honey
Sea salt
Freshly ground
  black pepper

This light vinaigrette is a classic French preparation. Serve this over assorted salad greens, or use it as a marinade and dressing for grilled vegetables.

In a small Mason jar, combine the olive oil, vinegar, lemon juice, thyme, mustard, and honey. Season with salt and pepper. Seal the lid and shake the jar to emulsify the ingredients. Refrigerate, covered, for up to 3 days. Bring out and let sit on the counter for 30 minutes to warm the oil before using. Shake again before pouring.

SUBSTITUTION TIP For a vegan version, use maple syrup, agave, or another sweetener instead of the honey.

PER SERVING (2 TABLESPOONS) Calories 149; Total Carbohydrates 1g; Sugar 1g; Total Fat 17g; Saturated Fat 2g; Sodium 45mg; Protein 0g; Fiber 0g

BALSAMIC
Vinaigrette

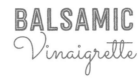

MAKES ¾ CUP ○ PREP TIME: 5 MINUTES

ALLERGEN-FREE
NUT-FREE
ONE POT
VEGAN

½ cup extra-virgin olive oil
¼ cup balsamic vinegar
1 tablespoon minced
  fresh basil
Sea salt, for seasoning
Freshly ground black
  pepper, for seasoning

If you can afford it, I recommend using a good-quality aged balsamic vinegar. If not, you can add a teaspoon of brown sugar or honey, if not serving as a vegan dish, to the dressing to soften the acerbic flavor of the vinegar.

1. In a small Mason jar, combine the olive oil, vinegar, and basil. Season with salt and pepper. Seal the lid and shake the jar to emulsify the ingredients.

2. Refrigerate, covered, for up to 3 days. Let the dressing sit at room temperature for 30 minutes to warm the oil before using. Shake again before pouring.

INGREDIENT TIP Add a hint of citrus to the dressing with the zest of one orange.

PER SERVING (2 TABLESPOONS) Calories 145; Total Carbohydrates 0g; Sugar 0g; Total Fat 17g; Saturated Fat 2g; Sodium 40mg; Protein 0g; Fiber 0g

MOROCCAN
Dressing

MAKES ¾ CUP ° PREP TIME: 5 MINUTES

DAIRY-FREE
EGG-FREE
NUT-FREE
ONE POT

½ cup extra-virgin olive oil
2 tablespoons red
  wine vinegar
2 tablespoons white
  wine vinegar
1 tablespoon minced
  fresh parsley
1 teaspoon minced garlic
1 teaspoon anchovy paste
1 teaspoon ground cumin
1 teaspoon ground paprika
Sea salt
Freshly ground
  black pepper

I like to serve this dressing over sturdy greens along with a generous handful of grape tomatoes and thinly sliced red onion.

1. In a small Mason jar, combine the olive oil, red wine vinegar, white wine vinegar, parsley, garlic, anchovy paste, cumin, and paprika. Season with salt and pepper.

2. Seal the lid and shake the jar to emulsify the ingredients. Refrigerate, covered, for up to 3 days. Bring out and let sit on the counter for 30 minutes to warm the oil before using. Shake again before pouring.

INGREDIENT TIP Find anchovy paste near the canned tuna at the grocery store. If the paste isn't available, buy whole anchovies in a tin and mince them finely with a chef's knife.

PER SERVING (2 TABLESPOONS) Calories 151; Total Carbohydrates 1g; Sugar 0g; Total Fat 18g; Saturated Fat 2g; Sodium 93mg; Protein 0g; Fiber 0g

SOY-GINGER
Dressing

MAKES ¾ CUP ° PREP TIME: 5 MINUTES

NUT-FREE
ONE POT
VEGAN

⅓ cup canola oil
2 tablespoons gluten-free
  soy sauce
1 tablespoon rice
  wine vinegar
1 tablespoon freshly
  squeezed lime juice
1 tablespoon toasted
  sesame oil
1 teaspoon minced
  peeled fresh ginger
1 teaspoon minced garlic
1 teaspoon brown sugar
Sea salt
Freshly ground
  black pepper

This dressing is especially good for serving with thinly sliced cabbage, romaine lettuce, cilantro, mint, and cucumber.

1. In a small Mason jar, combine the canola oil, soy sauce, vinegar, lime juice, sesame oil, ginger, garlic, and brown sugar.

2. Season with salt and pepper. Seal the lid and shake the jar to emulsify the ingredients. Refrigerate, covered, for up to 3 days.

INGREDIENT TIP A little toasted sesame oil goes a long way, so do not use it in place of the canola oil.

PER SERVING (2 TABLESPOONS) Calories 135; Total Carbohydrates 1g; Sugar 1g; Total Fat 14g; Saturated Fat 1g; Sodium 340mg; Protein 0g; Fiber 0g

AIOLI

DAIRY-FREE
NUT-FREE
ONE POT

1 egg yolk
1 teaspoon freshly
  squeezed lemon juice
1 small garlic
  clove, minced
2 tablespoons extra-virgin
  olive oil
⅓ cup canola oil

This garlicky Mediterranean-style mayonnaise is delicious served with oven fries or as a topping for fish. You can spice it up with a little cayenne pepper or add some fresh herbs.

1. In a small bowl, whisk the egg yolk, lemon juice, and garlic until integrated.

2. Whisking constantly, slowly drizzle in the olive oil a few drops at a time.

3. Continuing to whisk constantly to emulsify, slowly drizzle in the canola oil a few drops at a time until the mixture is thick and pale.

4. Refrigerate, covered, for up to 3 days.

INGREDIENT TIP Raw eggs come with a risk of foodborne illness. Do not serve to pregnant people or those with compromised immune systems.

PER SERVING (1 TABLESPOON) Calories 117; Total Carbohydrates 0g; Sugar 0g; Total Fat 13g; Saturated Fat 1g; Sodium 1mg; Protein 0g; Fiber 0g

THAI SWEET CHILI

Sauce

MAKES ABOUT 1 CUP ∘ PREP TIME: 5 MINUTES ∘ COOK TIME: 6 MINUTES

DAIRY-FREE
EGG-FREE
NUT-FREE
ONE POT
VEGETARIAN
MAKE ALLERGEN-FREE

½ cup rice vinegar
½ cup water
½ cup sugar
3 tablespoons gluten-free
  fish sauce
1 teaspoon minced garlic
2 Thai chiles, minced,
  or 2 teaspoons red
  pepper flakes
1½ tablespoons
  cornstarch

This sweet-and-sour sauce is perfect for dipping the Coconut-Crusted Shrimp (page 114). The aromas from the sauce as it cooks can be overpowering, but they will dissipate and the sauce will be delicious.

1. In a small saucepan over medium heat, combine the rice vinegar, water, sugar, fish sauce, garlic, and Thai chiles. Bring to a simmer and cook for 5 minutes.

2. Transfer 2 tablespoons of the liquid to a glass measuring cup and whisk in the cornstarch to make a slurry, making sure there are no lumps. Stir this slurry back into the pan and continue cooking for 1 to 2 minutes, continuing to stir until the sauce thickens.

3. Cool, cover, and refrigerate for up to 3 days.

COOKING TIP If you're serving this to kids, reduce the amount of chiles by half for a less spicy sauce.

SUBSTITUTION TIP To make this recipe allergen-free, omit the fish sauce and use 1 teaspoon of sea salt. There are some vegan fish sauce substitutes available in Asian markets, as well.

PER SERVING (2 TABLESPOONS) Calories 65; Total Carbohydrates 14g; Sugar 13g; Total Fat 0g; Saturated Fat 0g; Sodium 521mg; Protein 0g; Fiber 1g

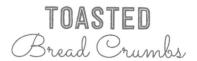

TOASTED
Bread Crumbs

MAKES 1 CUP • PREP TIME: 5 MINUTES • COOK TIME: 5 TO 7 MINUTES

ALLERGEN-FREE
DAIRY-FREE
NUT-FREE
VEGAN

4 slices gluten-free bread, torn into a few pieces
2 teaspoons extra-virgin olive oil
1 teaspoon minced garlic
1 teaspoon minced fresh herbs of your choice
Sea salt

Several recipes in this book, and beyond, call for bread crumbs. It's easy to make your own with gluten-free bread. Keep them plain and unsalted for use in other recipes. Or, toast them in a skillet or oven to make a delicious topping for salads or gluten-free pasta.

1. Preheat the oven to 325°F.

2. In a food processor, pulse the bread pieces at 1-second intervals until coarsely ground, making sure the bread doesn't form a dough ball. If using in other recipes, store the bread crumbs in a covered container for up to 5 days.

3. In a medium bowl, toss the bread crumbs with the olive oil, garlic, herbs, and a pinch salt.

4. Spread the crumbs on a rimmed baking sheet and toast for 5 to 7 minutes, or until gently browned. Cool before storing in a covered container for up to 5 days.

INGREDIENT TIP Gluten-free bread is expensive, so don't waste a crumb. Leave those crusts on! This is also a great way to use up bread that is going stale, or those pesky leftover bits of bread in the bag that aren't big enough for sandwiches. You can also start a collection of bread bits in the freezer just for this purpose, and pop them right into the food processor as needed.

PER SERVING (1 CUP) Calories 183; Total Carbohydrates 20g; Sugar 2g; Total Fat 11g; Saturated Fat 2g; Sodium 480mg; Protein 3g; Fiber 1g

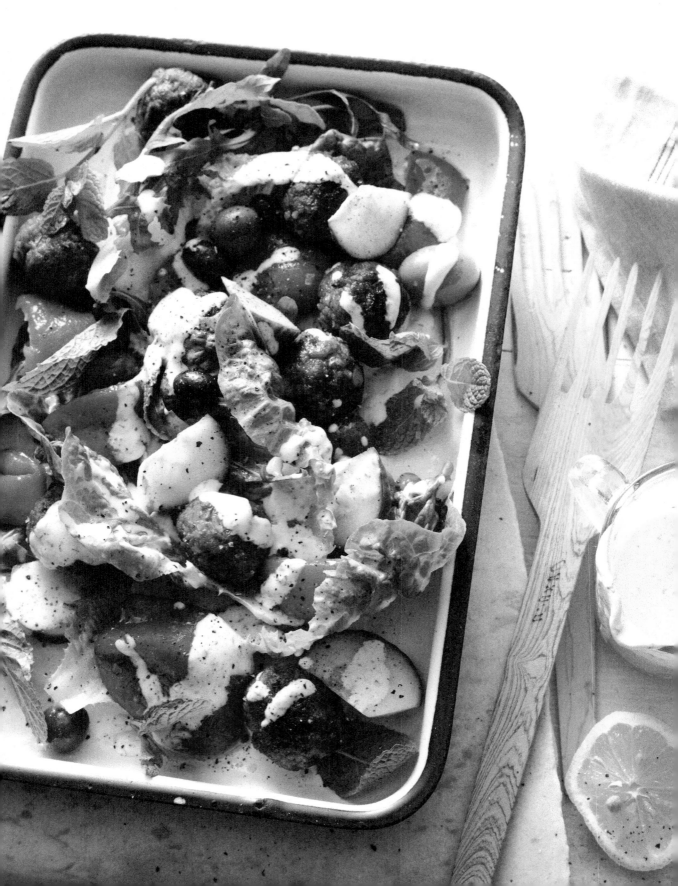

TEN TIPS
for Eating Out

Dining out at restaurants and at friends' houses can be a daunting experience, especially if you're newly gluten-free. Here are 10 tips to help you navigate with confidence.

1. If possible, choose restaurants that offer a gluten-free menu. You can usually find this out online.

2. Review menus ahead of time so you know a restaurant has something you can eat, or call ahead to ask if the chef can accommodate your dietary requirements.

3. Explain to your server or host that you have a medical condition and cannot eat gluten.

4. Explain to your server or host what kinds of foods contain gluten so they can help you find foods that are safe to eat.

5. Don't feel guilty sending servers to the kitchen to confirm that a dish is gluten-free or refusing certain foods at social functions. At the end of the day, you are responsible for your body and you have to live with it.

6. Beware of fried foods. Many foods cooked in a deep fryer are breaded. Even if the food you order is not breaded, it might be cooked in the same oil.

7. Ask twice about sauces—especially in restaurants. Many are thickened with flour.

8. If a dish arrives and you observe the presence of gluten (in the form of breading, soy sauce, or another telltale sign) send it back to the kitchen. It can be tempting to just eat it and deal with the consequences—especially for those without a life-threatening condition—but don't!

9. When dining with friends and family, offer to bring a dish to share.

10. Be gracious. Most people want to accommodate your needs, but sometimes they need a little guidance.

SUGGESTED MENUS

HEARTY BRUNCH
Perfect Hash Browns (page 42)
Sausage-Egg Muffin Cups (page 41)
Coffee Cake (page 48)
Orange juice and coffee

VEGETARIAN BRUNCH
Cheddar-Jalapeño Scones (page 51)
Vegetable Skillet Hash
    with Eggs (page 43)
Quinoa Fruit Salad (page 32)
Orange juice and coffee

CINCO DE MAYO PARTY
Baja Fish Tacos (page 108)
Avocado, Black Bean,
    and Quinoa Salad (page 95)
Baked Sweet Potato Fries (page 80)
Homemade margaritas

GAME DAY SMORGASBORD
Smoky Bacon and Roasted
    Corn Dip (page 86)
Crisp Potato Skins (page 81)
Crudités Platter (page 82)
Gluten-free beer

FAMILY BIRTHDAY DINNER
Panfried Crispy Chicken (page 132)
Mac 'n' Cheese (page 156)
No-Bake Cherry Cheesecake (page 195)

ELEGANT BIRTHDAY DINNER
Roasted Vegetables with
    Basil Oil (page 83)
New York Steak with
    Romesco Sauce (page 152)
Sour Cream Mashed Potatoes (page 96)
Flourless Chocolate Cake (page 202)

VEGAN FEAST
Crudités Platter (page 82)
Roasted Kabocha Squash
    over Quinoa (page 178)
Blackberry and Blueberry
    Crumble (page 203)

TAPAS NIGHT
Roasted Vegetables with
    Basil Oil (page 83)
Tortilla Española (page 158)
Prosciutto-Wrapped Dates (page 87)
Stuffed Mushrooms (page 89)

THE DIRTY DOZEN AND
The Clean Fifteen

A nonprofit and environmental watchdog organization called the Environmental Working Group (EWG) looks at data supplied by the US Department of Agriculture (USDA) and the Food and Drug Administration (FDA) about pesticide residues. Each year, it compiles a list of the lowest and highest pesticide loads found in commercial crops. You can use these lists to decide which fruits and vegetables to buy organic to minimize your exposure to pesticides and which conventional produce is considered safe enough to eat. This does not mean they are pesticide-free, though, so wash these (and all) fruits and vegetables thoroughly.

These lists change every year, so make sure you look up the most recent one before you fill your shopping cart. You'll find the most recent lists as well as a guide to pesticides in produce at EWG.org/FoodNews.

THE DIRTY DOZEN

Apples • Celery • Cherry tomatoes • Cucumbers • Grapes
Nectarines (imported) • Peaches • Potatoes • Snap peas (imported)
Spinach • Strawberries • Sweet bell peppers
(Kale/Collard greens • Hot peppers)*

*In addition to the dirty dozen, the EWG added two produce items contaminated with highly toxic organophosphate insecticides.

The Clean Fifteen

Asparagus • Avocados • Cabbage • Cantaloupes (domestic) •
Cauliflower • Eggplant • Grapefruit • Kiwi fruit •
Mangos • Onions • Papayas • Pineapples • Sweet corn •
Sweet peas (frozen) • Sweet potatoes

MEASUREMENT
Conversions

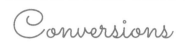

US STANDARD	US STANDARD (OUNCES)	METRIC (APPROXIMATE)
2 tablespoons	1 fl. oz.	30 mL
¼ cup	2 fl. oz.	60 mL
½ cup	4 fl. oz.	120 mL
1 cup	8 fl. oz.	240 mL
1½ cups	12 fl. oz.	355 mL
2 cups or 1 pint	16 fl. oz.	475 mL
4 cups or 1 quart	32 fl. oz.	1 L
1 gallon	128 fl. oz.	4 L

FAHRENHEIT (F)	CELSIUS (C) (APPROXIMATE)
250°F	120°C
300°F	150°C
325°F	165°C
350°F	180°C
375°F	190°C
400°F	200°C
425°F	220°C
450°F	230°C

VOLUME EQUIVALENTS (DRY)

US STANDARD	METRIC (APPROXIMATE)
¼ teaspoon	1 mL
½ teaspoon	2 mL
1 teaspoon	5 mL
1 tablespoon	15 mL
¼ cup	59 mL
⅓ cup	79 mL
½ cup	118 mL
1 cup	177 mL

WEIGHT EQUIVALENTS

US STANDARD	METRIC (APPROXIMATE)
½ ounce	15 g
1 ounce	30 g
2 ounces	60 g
4 ounces	115 g
8 ounces	225 g
12 ounces	340 g
16 ounces or 1 pound	455 g

RESOURCES AND REFERENCES

Resources

Beyond Celiac (www.beyondceliac.org): Advocacy group for people with celiac disease.

Celiac Disease Foundation (https://celiac.org): Nonprofit organization devoted to advocacy, education, and research.

Gluten Dude (http://glutendude.com): Gluten-free blog and supportive celiac community.

References

Abbas, Abul K., Andrew H. Lichtman, and Shiv Pillai. *Basic Immunology: Functions and Disorders of the Immune System*. 4th ed. Philadelphia: Saunders, 2012.

American College of Gastroenterology. "Diagnosis and Management of Celiac Disease." Accessed June 28, 2016. http://gi.org/guideline/diagnosis-and-management-of-celiac-disease.

Beyond Celiac. "Celiac Disease: Fast Facts" Accessed June 28, 2016. www.beyondceliac.org/celiac-disease/facts-and-figures.

Consumer Reports. "Arsenic in Your Food Investigated." Accessed July 18, 2016. http://www.consumerreports.org/cro/magazine/2012/11/arsenic-in-your-food/index.htm.

Four Winds Nutrition Carbohydrates and the Glycemic Index. Accessed June 29, 2016. www.webnat.com/articles/Glycemix.asp.

Lundin, Knut E.A. "Celiac Disease." In *Gastrointestinal Endoscopy Clinics of North America*. Retrieved from: www.researchgate.net/profile/Knut_Lundin/publication/232528784_Nonceliac_Gluten_Sensitivity/links/09e415098bbe37c05b000000.pdf. Accessed June 28, 2016. doi:10.1016/j.giec.2012.07.006.

Mayo Clinic. "Wheat Allergy." Accessed June 28, 2016. www.mayoclinic.org/diseases-conditions/wheat-allergy/basics/symptoms/con-20031834.

Midhagen, G., and C. Hallert. "High Rate of Gastrointestinal Symptoms in Celiac Patients Living on a Gluten-Free Diet: Controlled Study." *American Journal of Gastroenterology* 98, no. 9 (September 2003): 2023-6. Retrieved from: www.ncbi.nlm.nih.gov/pubmed/14499782.

Thompson, T. *"Wheat Starch, Gliadin, and the Gluten-Free Diet." Journal of the American Dietetic Association* 101, no. 12 (December 2001): 1456-9. Accessed June 28, 2016. www.ncbi.nlm.nih.gov/pubmed/11762742.

Tursi, A., G. Brandimarte, and G. Giorgetti. "High Prevalence of Small Intestinal Bacterial Overgrowth in Celiac Patients with Persistence of Gastrointestinal Symptoms After Gluten Withdrawal." *American Journal of Gastroenterology* 98, no. 4 (April 2003): 839-43. Retrieved from: www.ncbi.nlm.nih.gov/pubmed/12738465.

WebMD. "Leaky Gut Syndrome: What Is it?" Accessed June 28, 2016. Retrieved from: www.webmd.com/digestive-disorders/features/leaky-gut-syndrome.

RECICE INDEX

INDEX

ACKNOWLEDGMENTS

I am so grateful to Brad and Cole for their willingness to try new foods and for making sure the desserts taste good!

To Rich, for your love and endless support, for going gluten-free with me and the kids, and for always making sure I get time to surf.

To my mom, Lonnie, for encouraging me to bake from a young age.

To my editors at Callisto Media for pushing me to discover and create new recipes, and for your wisdom in shaping this manuscript into something I am proud of.

Special thanks to all of chefs who have graciously shared their culinary wisdom through books, blogs, television shows, and, especially, their food. I have learned so much from you that I can never call myself "self-taught." I'm especially grateful to the gluten-free pioneers who have taught me the essentials of gluten-free and grain-free baking, especially Annalise Roberts, Shauna James Ahern, and Danielle Walker.

ABOUT THE AUTHOR

Pamela Ellgen is a gluten-free food blogger and author of numerous books on cooking, nutrition, and fitness, including *Soup & Comfort, Baking Sheet Paleo,* and *Healthy Slow Cooker Cookbook for Two.* Her work has been published in Beachbody.com, *Huffington Post,* LIVESTRONG, *Darling* magazine, and Spinning.com. Pamela lives in Santa Barbara, California, with her husband and two sons. When she's not in the kitchen, she enjoys surfing and exploring the local farmers' market.

CPSIA information can be obtained
at www.ICGtesting.com
Printed in the USA
LVOW06s0314081117
554709LV00002B/2/P

9 781623 157845